homoeopathy for children

Gabrielle Pinto
and
Murray Feldman

# homoeopathy
# for children

a parent's guide to the treatment
of common childhood illnesses

index by
Mary Kirkness

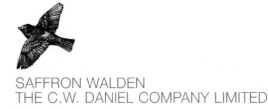

SAFFRON WALDEN
THE C.W. DANIEL COMPANY LIMITED

to the master healer H. W. L. Poonjaji

to the master homoeopath
Dr Vassilis Ghegas

First published in Great Britain by
Thorsons, an imprint of HarperCollins

This revised edition published in 2000 by
The C.W. Daniel Company Limited,
1 Church Path, Saffron Walden, Essex, CB10 1JP,
United Kingdom

ISBN 0 85207 337 2

Produced in association with
Book Production Consultants, plc,
25–27 High Street, Chesterton, Cambridge, CB4 1ND
Designed and typeset by Ward Partnership, Saffron Walden, Essex
Printed and bound by St Edmundsbury Press,
Bury St Edmunds, Suffolk

# contents

# acknowledgements

We wish to thank all those who have helped us to write this book – especially our clients, who have shared their lives with us, and our families, who have supported us while we have been working, teaching and writing. We also want to express our gratitude to the Homoeopaths who have taught and continue to teach us Homoeopathy.

We are most appreciative for the practical advice provided by Dr Richard Wynn for the medical section, and for Udi Eichler's contributions on psychotherapy. Martin Pollecoff assisted with the writing, and Bruce Owen came to the rescue when the computers started misbehaving – thanks to you both. Thanks must also go to Dr Roger Morrison for taking time out from an extremely busy schedule to write the Foreword.

We also wish to thank the Homoeopaths Laurie Dack, Susan Gimbel and Iain Marrs for their case study contributions and for reading through the manuscript. Thanks, too, go to Karen Dawson, Imogen Budd and Kim Boutillier for their endless patience and support, and to Mitra Feldman, who provided Murray with his first experience of prescribing for a child.

Special thanks must go to our editor, Erica Smith, who encouraged us from the beginning to write this book.

# foreword

In recent years there have been many excellent introductory texts on homoeopathy. These texts have often included some information about home health care. However, none of these books has addressed the full needs of families with children. This present work by Murray Feldman and Gabrielle Pinto answers this need perfectly.

The authors, both highly respected practitioners and teachers of homoeopathy, have collaborated to make this book both complete and easily comprehensible. It covers almost every kind of health condition. Nothing is left unexplained. The book guides the parent on how to select, administer, store and evaluate the homoeopathic medicines. In addition it explains the reasons for each health problem and the warning signals which indicate a need for professional evaluation. Each chapter is carefully crafted to walk the parents through every concern.

The final part of the book goes through the most common constitutional types, giving a clear picture of each remedy. This will help the parent prepare for an interview with a homoeopath by indicating the depth and areas of interest for the practitioner. Also, the constitutional pictures provide a context for the parent to understand the full workings of homoeopathy.

This is a book which fills a great need in our profession and society. It is a well-organized and practical book on the most effective type of alternative medicine which can be used at home. Every family should use this book!

Dr Roger Morrison

# introduction

How many of us have stood and watched our children suffer from repeated earaches, colds and fevers, only to see them given antibiotics over and over again and reassured that nothing is seriously wrong? Sometimes we have been told that 'nothing can be done. You just have to wait.'

This book is meant for those of you who really want to know if there is an alternative to this. An alternative that is safe, non-toxic and effective.

Homoeopathy is one of the oldest and most accepted forms of natural medicine. It was discovered almost 200 years ago, although the advent of modern drugs meant that interest in it waned considerably during the first part of this century. However, enthusiasm for homoeopathy is now undergoing a tremendous resurgence throughout the world. One of the major reasons for this is the realization that orthodox drugs are not fulfilling our original hopes. New strains of bacteria, an increase in chronic disease, and the side-effects of certain drugs have led people to turn to homoeopathy. This is not meant to belittle the advances made and help given by orthodox medicine – but drugs are not always the only answer.

There are people who take pain-killers for every ache, and sleeping pills or anti-depressants at the slightest hint of tension or sleeplessness. Although these drugs definitely have short-term value, they offer only temporary and at times imperfect relief. The continual use of drugs can weaken the body's own resistance, leading to increased reliance or addiction and making a complete cure more difficult.

Homoeopathy, on the other hand, is 'holistic'. That is to say, it treats the whole person – the individual who is sick – rather than just his or her symptoms. For this reason there is no one medicine indicated for everyone affected by a certain illness. Although they may have exactly the same disease, different people need different remedies.

Before prescribing a remedy, a homoeopath will take into account the patient's demeanour, emotional state, and how he responds, either mentally or physically, to the stresses in his life.

In our experience as homoeopaths we have been delighted to see how quickly children respond to homoeopathic medicine. In adults the natural picture of disease is often distorted by their past history of emotional trauma or over-use of drugs. Even birth control pills can upset the hormonal cycle and alter healthy bodily functioning. Children, on the other hand, have not usually the same history of taking orthodox drugs for their symptoms, and *they reveal their symptoms spontaneously* just by being themselves. Their natural capacity for health, healing and happiness has not yet been reduced or distorted by over-medication or by their own feelings, beliefs and anxieties about life.

People who say that homoeopathic medicines act by suggestion need only watch how a baby responds to homoeopathy. It is wonderful to see a child saved from the need to have his tonsils removed or tubes put in his ears by the use of well-chosen remedies.

## Using Homoeopathy to Treat Simple Illnesses

This book is intended primarily as a self-help guide. It is meant to support you in actively participating in your child's health during bouts of minor acute ailments such as coughs and colds, and non-life-threatening conditions that require first-aid treatment.

We have tried to explain the subject of homoeopathy simply, to make it easy and effective to use. It is aimed at the reader who knows nothing or very little about homoeopathy.

This book is also meant to introduce you to the idea that homoeopathy can be extremely effective in treating chronic diseases such as mumps and measles, and problems such as hyperactivity, bedwetting and the after-effects of some kind of emotional stress. You will not be told how to treat these chronic conditions yourself, but merely helped to gain an understanding of how homoeopathy may be used by a professional homoeopath as a cure for these problems. You will discover the most commonly indicated remedies for such problems, by way of introduction to the science of homoeopathy.

This book is not meant to make you a homoeopath or to teach you how to treat long-term chronic diseases. Nor can this short book take the place of professional medical diagnosis or advice; we would always recommend that you seek professional help when dealing with severe acute illnesses. If you are the least bit uncertain or worried in any situation, see your doctor for a diagnosis. In fact, doing so will help you to use this book more effectively.

Parents are naturally anxious when their children are ill. It takes great courage to consider using homoeopathy instead of antibiotics or other drugs. Homoeopathic remedies are *gentle and safe*. So even if you do not get it right the first time, you are not putting your child at risk. We recommend that you start by using this book only for minor problems, to build your confidence. Once you have witnessed your child recover from a simple illness such as a cold or fever, you will be in a much better position to treat other complaints and even to consider incorporating homoeopathic treatment into your family's life from now on.

We are confident that you will be amazed by the benefits of homoeopathy on your child and will be inspired to learn more about this wonderful system of healing.

## How to Use This Book

Chapter 1 explains how to 'take your child's case' – that is, collect all the relevant information so you can decide which homoeopathic remedy will be most effective. This chapter also briefly outlines the important homoeopathic principles you will need to be familiar with. **Important homoeopathic terms used throughout the book are defined here and in the Glossary** (*see page 201*). We would also recommend that you read Chapter 2 on the history and philosophy behind homoeopathic medicine. This will help you in taking a case and prescribing.

The Treatments part of the book is broken into three sections:

1  First aid (Chapter 4)
2  Common illnesses and everyday complaints (Chapter 5)
3  Contagious childhood diseases (Chapter 6)

Having chosen which of these three chapters you need, compare your child's symptoms to the symptoms outlined under the different homoeopathic remedies listed there. The symptoms printed in **bold** type are the most significant ones.

All the symptoms listed under a remedy do not have to be present for a diagnosis to be correct. Three marked symptoms, relating to the child himself (his emotional and mental state) and not just to his illness, are usually enough for you to be confident that you have chosen well.

If you are unsure about whether you have chosen the right remedy, look at the **Materia Medica** section (Chapter 10). This will help clarify your options. The modalities (those circumstances that make your child's symptoms better or worse), typical behaviour and one or two characteristic symptoms (again, peculiar to the child, not the disease) are more important than the symptoms of the illness itself, which are common to every child who has that particular problem.

After you identify the correct remedy, give it to your child as instructed. Give only one remedy at a time. If your child is suffering from two complaints at the same time, treat the most urgent or severe one first, before dealing with the other.

For each disease or condition we have provided a reliable guideline on the potency to use and how often to repeat it. Repetition is always guided by the intensity of the problem. You may, therefore, find it helpful to read the section on **Selection of Potency and Repetition** in Chapter 3.

Chapter 8, on **Emotional Development**, is included for your own information. Homoeopathy can often be very effective for these types of problems, but we recommend you also seek professional help.

Please note that throughout this book we have alternated the use of 'he' and 'she' when referring to a child.

# section one

## what is
## homoeopathy?

chapter one

# taking your child's case

To understand what is troubling your child so you can treat him with the correct homoeopathic remedy, you need to be able to recognize whether his problem calls for simple first-aid measures, is an acute condition, or is chronic. This book can help you with first-aid cases and acute conditions; chronic diseases, however, will require the help of a professional homoeopath or your family doctor.

### First Aid Cases

Homoeopathy has a good track record with bruises, stings, sprains, wounds, fractures, skin abrasions, burns and other such injuries, which generally have an external cause and are not related to a child's history or susceptibility (that is, each person's own unique response to disease). Conditions such as these may, however, also need additional care. A broken bone, for example, will of course need a cast as well as the required homoeopathic remedy.

### Acute Diseases

Acute diseases are those which have a definite beginning and end, and happen only occasionally. Frequently these diseases may have an obvious cause, as in the case of food poisoning or catching a cold after getting caught in the rain. All childhood diseases (such as measles and mumps) fall under this category too, as do flu, coughs, earache and other such complaints. With acute diseases we start to see a variety of individual symptoms; they differ in this from cases requiring first-aid treatment.

Simple acute disease can often be treated at home quite effectively with homoeopathic remedies. Acute diseases usually disappear of their own accord over a period of time, but the proper homoeopathic treatment will help ease suffering and prevent complications.

Having said this, some acute diseases – such as pneumonia – can be life-threatening. These fall outside the scope of this book and need professional help.

## Chronic Diseases

Chronic diseases have several distinguishing characteristics. They tend to recur persistently (as in the case of some types of earache, flu, coughs, colds, tonsillitis and skin problems). Although they may seem acute, the fact that these conditions come back over and over again makes them chronic.

Conditions that get worse as the years go by are also termed chronic. A child may be born with a chronic disorder of this kind, although sometimes it has no apparent or definite beginning.

Chronic diseases can also often start after a severe acute disease or a strong emotional trauma. There is a phrase in homoeopathy for such conditions: 'never been well since'.

Chronic diseases show no tendency to go away of their own accord, like acute ones do. They are far more complicated to treat and definitely require the skills of a professional homoeopath, as they do involve a child's susceptibility.

We recommend that, if you feel unsure about what is troubling your child, you contact a professional homoeopath or your medical doctor immediately.

## How to Take Your Child's Case

In homoeopathy the term 'symptoms' has a very broad meaning, in that any and all recent changes from the healthy state to illness are taken into account. Indications such as fever, pulse rate, perspiration, changes in bowel habits and urine are taken into account, but more important are the symptoms that are unique to your particular child.

Each child must be treated not just for a disease but as an individual case of that disease. For example, the symptoms of flu are well known: aching, fever, tiredness, weakness. But while a child may have these common flu symptoms, he may also want nothing to drink, for you to stay near him, and to be kept quite warm; another will be extremely thirsty, dislike company and be unable to tolerate heat; a third may feel chilly, be weepy and keep asking for a cool drink. These, then, are examples of the symptoms of the sick child, the individual case of the disease. It is to these symptoms that homoeopathy attaches most importance.

Each of these three children will need a different remedy for the same disease, because their individual symptoms are different. What are the symptoms that make your child's disease unique? This is what you need to find out in each situation.

As well as physical symptoms, disease can also produce mental and emotional ones. Your normally happy and independent son may suddenly become clingy and irritable; your very affectionate daughter may suddenly want only to be left alone. It is important to take these types of changes into account when deciding which remedy to use. In fact, homoeopaths sometimes base their prescriptions almost entirely on these changes alone.

You may also notice a change in your child's appetite: he may suddenly refuse to touch a food that was his favourite, or he may demand a food he used to hate the sight of; a normally thirsty child may now seem never to want a drink at all.

The circumstances that make your child's condition better or worse are called *modalities*; they are of great importance. A child with colic may improve if you give him a hot water bottle. A child with fever may feel better with the window open, or may only stop crying if you carry him about. Your child may have a sore throat that improves if he is given a warm drink. The child who never usually complains about the cold now cannot get warm enough. These are a few examples of modalities; taking note of them can help you choose the right remedy for your child.

Another useful indication can be the way in which your child describes a pain or sensation. He may express it as cramping, burning, heavy, bruised, or 'as if …' ('as if a ball is in my tummy' or 'as if a tight bandage is around my head'). These descriptions are very useful and must not be forgotten when you are looking for a remedy or reporting symptoms to your homoeopath.

To identify your child's symptoms effectively you will often have to make careful observations, particularly if your child is too young or too unwell to talk to you. You may find the following list of value to help you find the information you need.

1  *Causation* – this can be very important. Did the problem start, for example, after your child got wet? Are the days warm and nights cold? Did your child get ill after being out in a strong, dry, cold wind? These are indications for a particular set of remedies.

2  *Temperature* – check if it is high or low. If it seems to fluctuate throughout the day, make a note of what time of day it changes.

3  *Breathing* – notice if it is affected and how.

4  *Skin colour* – look for any changes, for example flushing, paleness, or red cheeks.

5  *Perspiration* – is your child perspiring more (or less) than usual? Does his perspiration smell differently than normal? Is he perspiring from areas of his body not normally affected?

6  *Temperament and expression* – is your child irritable, weepy, anxious, fearful or indifferent? How does he respond to affection, to company?

7  *Delirium* – is the child delirious? – if so, what is he saying?

8  *Voice* – what is his voice like? – weak, croaky, faint, etc.

9  *Location* – where is the pain?

10  *Sensation* – how does he describe the pain?

11  *Better/Worse* – what makes him and/or the pain better or worse?

12  *Appetite and thirst* – is the child hungry or thirsty? If so, what does he want to eat/drink? Does he want hot or cold drinks/ food?

13  *Energy* – is he just lying there or watching TV? Is he too ill even to play with his favourite toys, or is he jumping about?

14 *Covering* – does he want the covers on or off, the windows open or shut?

15 *Time* – what time of the day or night is he worse or better?

16 *Unusual symptoms* – is there anything unusual about your child's behaviour or something that you would not expect in the disease he has? Symptoms that seem strange, peculiar or unusual to you are also of value. Examples of this might be a child with a high temperature who nevertheless seems not to be thirsty at all, or a child with an abscess who feels better if you touch it.

17 *What is the medical diagnosis?*

## For Babies and Very Young Children

Carefully watch what babies do. If they continually put their hands to their ears, they may have ear problems. If they draw their knees up to their abdomen, they may have colic. Do they grasp at their throat or their head? Do they cry out before they urinate or pass a stool? All these observations will tell you a great deal about the possible location and nature of your child's illness. Adults tell us about their problems; children often show them to us.

# chapter two

# history and philosophy of homoeopathy

## History and the Law of Similars

If Dr Samuel Hahnemann (1755–1843) had kept to his ideas regarding nutrition and hygiene, he would have been recognized as one of the great reformers in medical history. Instead he discovered homoeopathy, and was considered one of medicine's heretics.

Hahnemann qualified as a medical practitioner in Germany in 1779. During his years as a general physician he grew disillusioned with the profession, before finally quitting to research 'a way less cruel'.

At the time, the method of prescribing drugs was haphazard; poisonous potions were often administered. Disease was regarded as a consequence of bad blood and patients were regularly leeched, purged and bled.

To be able to continue to support his family, Hahnemann began translating foreign works of chemistry. He became obsessed with the idea of finding a universal principle underlying the nature of disease, and how to administer medicines in order to bring about a safe, effective cure.

In 1790, whilst translating an essay by the famous Scottish physician William Cullen on the use of Peruvian Bark in certain types of fevers, Hahnemann was struck by something Cullen reported: the bark worked because of its bitter and astringent properties.

Hahnemann knew that other medicines had these same properties, so he could not accept Cullen's theory as to why Peruvian Bark had effected this cure. Hahnemann decided to take large amounts of the bark himself; within a couple of days he had developed the symptoms of a malaria-like fever. This was the birth of homoeopathy, which has as one of its main precepts 'like treats like'. The bark, when taken in large amounts by a healthy person, produced symptoms similar to those of malaria; if taken by a malaria sufferer in small amounts, he would recover. This became known as the *law of similars*, the basic principle of homoeopathic treatment.

## Testing on Healthy People

Hahnemann wanted to test his concept and bravely took other medicines of the day. He also administered them to his students, his medical colleagues, and other healthy people who were interested in his theory.

He carefully recorded every change that took place in his volunteers, noting the type of pains they had, how each substance affected the stool, the urine, the menstrual flow, the desire for particular foods, even the person's reaction to weather changes. He observed how each new substance affected the mind, the emotions, the sleep – in short, the whole human being.

These extremely comprehensive records became known in homoeopathy as the *provings*. Hahnemann collected these provings into books known as the *Materia Medica*.

When sick people came with symptoms similar to those listed in the provings of a certain substance, Hahnemann gave them that substance in small amounts. It worked; people recovered. Hahnemann called this branch of healing homoeopathy, from the Greek words *homoios* (like or similar) and *pathos* (suffering).

Let us give you an example of a 'proving'. Let's use an everyday occurrence that we are all aware of: cutting up an onion. What happens when we cut or eat a raw onion? Our eyes sting or water, our nose may run with a burning discharge, we may start to sneeze. Some people may be so affected that they have difficulty breathing. These symptoms, when recorded, are 'the provings of onion'.

When a person comes to a homoeopath with a cold, and demonstrating the above symptoms, he or she will be prescribed homoeopathically prepared onion (*Allium sativa*).

In spite of much opposition from some doctors and pharmacists, homoeopathy's popularity grew rapidly during Hahnemann's lifetime. Hospitals and colleges spread throughout Europe and North America. By the end of the last century about 15 per cent of all physicians in North America were homoeopaths.

This growth in the practice of homoeopathy was only checked by the advent of antibiotics and other 'wonder' drugs. In the years following the Second World War there was a widespread belief that modern science could banish all ills, including ignorance and poverty. Today we are much more aware of the possible and real side-effects of many of our discoveries, and so the gentle and safe practice of homoeopathy has once more enjoyed a resurgence.

In India homoeopathy has equal recognition with orthodox medicine and with ayurveda, and there are hospitals and colleges of homoeopathy throughout the country supported by the government. In Britain the Royal family have a homoeopathic physician on their staff.

## How Homoeopathic Remedies Are Prepared

Hahnemann was not entirely satisfied with having discovered the concept of 'similar medicine'. Even though people recovered with his homoeopathic treatments, some patients got worse before they got better.

He wondered if the doses he was prescribing were too large. He decided to dilute the substances, and found that they still worked, though still not as well as he'd hoped.

He now had an inspiration. He decided to dilute, then vigorously shake the homoeopathic preparations rather than stir them. To his surprise, and certainly to his satisfaction, the results were better than ever. This new methodology helped to speed up patients' recovery.

This was astonishing to Hahnemann. Here were substances that when highly diluted reached a point where they stopped having any effect, but which when shaken (or as he called it, *succussed*) brought about cure. Medicines prepared in this way became known as *potentized* remedies. This method of dilution and succussion became the basis for the preparation of homoeopathic medicines to this day. All remedies are prepared by homoeopathic pharmacies according to the strict specifications described by Hahnemann.

After much experimentation Hahnemann standardized two scales of preparation. One scale is known as the decimal scale, the other as the centesimal scale. Within both these scales a remedy's strength is listed by a number (6, 12 or 30) following the name of the remedy. The decimal scale is indicated by an X, as in 6X or 12X; the centesimal scale is classified with either a C, CH, or nothing following the potency number.

These numbers represent the extent to which the remedy is diluted and succussed. The higher the number, the less of the actual material amount of the substance is present in the remedy.

As a result of this process Hahnemann was able to make use of very minute amounts of various substances. This allowed him to experiment with a variety of sources from the animal, plant and mineral kingdoms. It even allowed him to use poisonous substances without any toxic effect.

Potentization is one of the great mysteries of homoeopathy. However, it is important to understand that what makes a remedy homoeopathic is not the potentization, but the fact that it is given according to the law of similars.

Potentization has caused many people to dismiss homoeopathy. To the logically minded doctor or scientist, it seems impossible that something so very diluted can trigger a specific healing reaction. With the latest advances in quantum physics it seems inevitable that this mystery will be solved in the not too distant future.

## What is Health?

What do we consider the signs of good health to be in our children?

For the homoeopath, health is the ability to adapt easily to environmental changes on a mental, emotional and physical level.

When we look at the eyes of a healthy child we see a brightness, a vitality, an innate joy. Naturally we use such terms as 'radiant health'.

It is the vitality of our children that we instinctively notice when they start to become ill. One child has a glazed look, feels weak and is slightly off her food, even though there is nothing specifically wrong. Another child has a runny nose and a cough, yet her appetite and energy levels are normal, and her eyes are bright. Which child do we worry about the most? The one whose vitality is low even though there is no specific disease, or the 'sick' one whose vitality remains high and undiminished? Homoeopaths worry more about the child with the low vitality.

Hahnemann recognized this vitality, which we have not yet been able to measure, as an inherent aspect of life. He observed through his method of preparing remedies that this vitality could be released. This vitality animates every living substance and person. Hahnemann called this unseen yet evident energetic factor in your child, which is affected in ill health and which can be stimulated by homoeopathic remedies, the *Vital Force*.

## What is Disease?

To the homoeopath, disease is an imbalance which affects the whole person. First his or her vitality is affected, perhaps as a result of exposure to poor weather, lack of sleep, continuous stress or a variety of other factors. When this imbalance persists, symptoms 'localize' in specific areas such as the tonsils, neck muscles or stomach. This localization is usually considered to be 'the disease'. However, homoeopaths see this localization as the 'result' of the disease. The true disease, the imbalance, was there prior to the localization. Disease manifests itself by signs or symptoms on the mental, emotional and/or physical level. It is a state of disharmony when the ability to adjust is lacking and the freedom to express our creativity is limited. The presence and intensity of symptoms are, therefore, related to the body's ability or inability to adjust to changes in the environment.

### Susceptibility to Illness

Every individual reacts differently to the same situation, even to the same bacteria. One child exposed to wet, cold weather will suffer no ill-effects; another will come down with a cold for a day; a third will suffer for two days; yet another will get bronchitis. These varying reactions are the result of each individual's unique susceptibility or response to the external 'cause'. The 'quality' of someone's susceptibility is affected by many factors, including diet, the amount of stress in his or her life, and inherited tendencies.

In orthodox medicine, drugs are used to kill bacteria or subdue inflammation – in other words to reduce the symptoms. The purpose of a homoeopathic remedy is to stimulate the vitality, to increase the body's own resistance to disease and capacity to heal itself. Homoeopathy treats your child's susceptibility. In this it differs markedly from orthodox drug treatment.

### What is Cure?

For a homoeopath, cure is more than simply the removal of the local pain. It seeks to make the whole person feel better. This is why it is important to be able to tell if true cure is taking place. The way of observing this was formulated by a German homoeopathic physician, Constantine Hering. It is known as Hering's Law of Direction of Cure. It applies particularly to chronic diseases, but may also be observed in acute diseases.

1  Disease gets better from the inside out.
   *This can be seen in two ways: First, your child starts to feel
   better in herself. An increase in energy often precedes an
   improvement in physical symptoms. In acute diseases the child
   may fall asleep soon after taking a remedy. She may feel more
   lively, with an improvement in her mood. These are good
   indications that she is getting better even if the pain, cough, etc. is
   still present.*

2 Cure takes place from above downwards.
  *An example of this would be in the case of a rash. It would clear up on the face before it cleared up on the feet.*
3 Cure takes place in reverse order of appearance.
  *In chronic disease, symptoms that a child had previously may return as the child starts to get better.*

chapter three

# selecting, taking and storing remedies

## Selecting the Right Potency and Repetition

One of the most important things to take into account, when choosing which potency of a particular remedy to use, is the degree of similarity between the 'provings' of the remedy and your child's symptoms.

The more precisely the remedy and your child's symptoms 'match', the higher the potency you can use. However, for those of you who have little experience with homoeopathy, the 6C, 12C and 30C potencies are the best to use. Unless otherwise mentioned in the specific sections on the different diseases, it is best not to use remedies in potencies higher than 30, and you should only use 30 when you are quite sure that you have got the 'similimum' – that is, the remedy that precisely covers the major symptoms.

One of Hahnemann's key rules was to use the minimum amount, that is, as few doses as possible. Generally, the more intense the acute sickness, the more you will need to repeat the dose. In very high fevers or where there is very intense pain, a dose might need to be given every half hour to every one and a half hours before there is lasting relief. Very occasionally the dose might have to be administered even more frequently than this. In most cases, however, one dose every two to five hours is sufficient.

If after one to three doses there is marked relief, stop giving the remedy; your child will probably continue to get better. If the relief plateaus for another day or your child starts to relapse, repeat the remedy. If the relief is noticeable but slight, give two or three more doses, lengthening the time between repeat doses as your child continues to improve.

Usually if there is no relief whatsoever after three or four doses, the remedy is not correct. Remember that relief can take the form of an improvement in your child's disposition or his ability to get some rest rather than in his physical symptoms of pain or discomfort.

If the symptoms change completely you may need to follow the first remedy with a second one that matches the new symptoms. For most acute diseases treated by this book, one remedy will usually be sufficient. Rarely will more than two be required.

**Remember: do not give your child two different remedies at the same time.**

If you give the remedy in the late afternoon, repeat it two or three times; there should be signs of relief by the next morning if the remedy is correct. There will usually be relief within 12 to 24 hours for most of the conditions mentioned in this book. During this period your child should not get worse, although his recovery may be slow. The childhood infectious diseases will usually go through their different stages, but complications and unnecessary distress may be averted by the correct prescribing of homoeopathic medicines.

Do not be in a hurry to switch to another remedy so long as your child is improving, however slowly. Do not get impatient and expect a 'miracle' cure, although they do sometimes happen. Sometimes the most difficult person to treat is your own child, because no parent wants his or her child to suffer and it is natural for you to want any remedy to have an immediate effect. But stick with a remedy and let it run its course; it will work if you have chosen well and can be patient.

**HOW TO TAKE AND STORE REMEDIES**

1  Make sure your child puts nothing in his mouth (no food, no drink, not even toothpaste) for at least 20 minutes before or after taking the remedy (strong odours such as those of camphor, eucalyptus or perfume can counteract a remedy).

2  Let the remedy dissolve on or under the tongue (do not drink anything to help it dissolve). This will allow the remedy to be absorbed quickly and easily.

3  Tablets or granules should not be touched, but poured into the cap of the bottle and put directly into the mouth.

4  Remedies should be stored in their original containers and kept away from bright light, heat, and strong smells (including perfumes). Do not keep them in the kitchen or the bathroom. If stored correctly, remedies will last indefinitely.

Remedies are available as liquid tinctures, tablets, or granules (small, round, sugar-like crystals). Granules are much more suitable for babies as they dissolve almost immediately. Your homoeopathic chemist will be able to advise you on how many granules, tablets or drops of a remedy will equal one dose.

Granules and tablets have a lactose or sucrose base, with drops of the remedy (in liquid form) added on top by the homoeopathic manufacturer. They taste sweet so babies and children find them easy to take. If your child has a lactose intolerance or diabetes, the remedies can be prepared in a liquid mixed with water and a small amount of alcohol.

## What to Avoid During Treatment

During homoeopathic treatment, avoid the use of camphor, menthol, eucalyptus, mint and coffee. Any of these substances – which are often found in cough syrups, Tiger Balm, nasal sprays and lip balms – can counteract the effects of homoeopathic treatment.

## Home Care Kit

The following is a suggestion of the remedies you may need for everyday care. The first six remedies listed are essential for your first aid kit. Add the remaining remedies when you can.

Choose either 6C, 12C or 30C potency. The 6C or 12C is a good potency to start with, unless another potency is specified for a given disease in the relevant section of this book.

You can have a kit made up for you at the pharmacies listed in the Useful Addresses chapter (*see page 205*), or at your local chemist if it stocks homoeopathic remedies.

More remedies are listed under specific sections in this book; your homoeopath may also recommend additional ones.

**ESSENTIAL FIRST AID REMEDIES:**

| | |
|---|---|
| *Aconite* | mental shock with fear; ailments after a severe fright |
| *Arnica montana* | bruises; problems after falls, accidents and injuries |
| *Arsenicum album* | vomiting and diarrhoea; food poisoning |
| *Hypericum* | injuries to nerves, fingertips and toes |
| *Ledum* | puncture wounds; insect stings |
| *Rhus toxicodendron* | sprains and strains |

**REMEDIES TO BE ADDED WHEN POSSIBLE:**

| | |
|---|---|
| *Apis mellifica* | *Hepar sulphuris* |
| *Belladonna* | *Ipecacuanha* |
| *Bryonia* | *Mercurius vivus* |
| *Cantharis* | *Pulsatilla* |
| *Chamomilla* | *Ruta graveolens* |
| *Dulcamara* | *Sulphur* |
| *Ferrum phosphoricum* | *Symphytum* |
| *Gelsemium* | *Urtica urens* |

**CREAMS FOR EXTERNAL USE:**

*Calendula* cream                         *Arnica* cream
Homoeopathic burn cream   *Urtica urens* cream (if
                                              homoeopathic burn cream is not
                                              available)
Hypercal ointment

**TINCTURES FOR EXTERNAL APPLICATION:**

*Calendula*
*Hypericum*
*Urtica urens*

Please read the **Materia Medica** section for a more detailed account
of these remedies.

# section two

treating your child
with homoeopathy

# chapter four

# homoeopathic first aid

Homoeopathy has a wide variety of remedies to suit many emergencies. A good knowledge of them will help alleviate pain and distress when your child has been injured.

Certain emergency situations will require immediate medical attention, which may mean going to the casualty department (emergency room) at the hospital. Correctly chosen, homoeopathic remedies will be effective while waiting for assistance or to help in the healing process afterwards.

Over the years we have consistently been told by parents how surprised they and their doctors were at the rapid recovery their children have made after homoeopathic treatment.

It is important to remember that, if the effects of an injury last longer than is normal, or if new complaints develop after an injury, chronic treatment may be needed. These would be examples of 'never been well since' conditions.

## Animal Bites and Puncture Wounds

### Hypericum

- ◆ **puncture wounds**
- ◆ **nerve damage**, especially with **shooting pains**
- ◆ animal bites

*Hypericum* would be the second remedy (after *Ledum*) in the treatment of puncture wounds and/or animal bites. It can be used internally or externally. *Hypericum* is useful if the nerves (such as in the fingertips) are also damaged after an injury involving a tack, nail or similar. Animal bites fall into this category, as they are punctures to the skin. If *Ledum* has been given and a red streak goes up the injured limb, or if pain starts shooting along the nerve pathways, *Hypericum* must now be given. It will help relieve the pains and heal the wound and nerves.

*Potency and Repetition*

*Hypericum 30* can be given every hour for three or four doses to help alleviate shooting pains. If the pains are not shooting, one dose of *Ledum 30* every hour for four doses can be given, followed by one dose of *Hypericum* every three hours for three doses.

### Ledum

- ◆ **puncture wounds** from nails, wire, etc.
- ◆ animal bites

*Ledum* prevents wounds from becoming septic and is the first remedy to be considered for a puncture to the skin. If your child gets a tack in her foot or hand, or steps on a nail, she will benefit from *Ledum*. Please also read *Hypericum* (above) for help with these types of wounds.

*Potency and Repetition*

*Ledum 30* can be given every half hour for three or four doses.

**EXTERNAL AND COMMON-SENSE MEASURES**

1  All puncture wounds should first be washed and soaked for
   10 minutes in a lotion of 15 drops *Hypericum* mother tincture
   (a solution made from the base plant soaked in alcohol) in
   half a glass of boiled or mineral water. The wound should
   then be covered with either *Hypercal* or *Calendula* ointment
   and a plaster.
2  If the bleeding is profuse and needs to be stopped, apply
   pressure with a cloth soaked in *Hypericum* lotion.

**WHEN TO SEEK PROFESSIONAL HELP**

The most serious worry with these types of wounds is tetanus.

Both *Ledum* and *Hypericum* are said to be tetanus preventatives.
You must really make up your own mind on this. Certainly if you
decide to get a tetanus injection, these remedies will help alleviate the
pain and stimulate the healing process. The other concern is the
possibility of contracting rabies after an animal bite. Medical help
must be sought immediately where this is a possibility.

## Bruises

Arnica montana

◆ **bruises or pain caused by blows, falls, accidents**
◆ problems resulting from over-exertion

This is a wonderful remedy for any type of injury or accident,
especially where there is bruising or the potential for bruising. It also
deals effectively with shock caused by injuries. In the provings,
*Arnica* produced the following symptom: 'Go away, there's nothing
wrong with me.' When a person has an accident, is this not one of
the first things she often says? *Arnica* helps deal with the physical
and mental trauma. It also helps heal broken capillaries. You will be
pleasantly surprised at its effects.

This remedy is also used for conditions where there is a bruised,
aching feeling after extreme exertion.

*Potency and Repetition*

*Arnica 30C* depending on the severity. At first it can be given every half hour for three doses, then every two to three hours for a few days. If the bruising is not so serious, administer one dose every hour for three or four doses. When given after an accident when the child needs rest, or when there is long-term bruising, one dose three times a day for a week is usually sufficient.

## Ledum

- ◆ **bruises and/or swellings that persist after *Arnica* has been given**
- ◆ especially indicated **if the bruised area feels cold**

*Ledum* is the remedy to give for a bruise or the swelling accompanying a bruise as a result of an injury when *Arnica* has ceased to work. Bruises that can be helped by *Ledum* may feel cold to the touch, and often improve if you apply a cold compress. Even if this symptom is not present, however, *Ledum* can still be prescribed.

*Potency and Repetition*

One dose of 30C three times a day for three or four days.

## Burns and Scalds

Minor burns can be successfully treated with homoeopathy, but we advise you to look out for the following factors in the case of children's burns:

1  What caused the burn?: Was it a faulty electrical appliance, hot objects and liquids, chemicals or fire?
2  Where is the burn?
3  How great an area of skin has been burned?
4  Which degree is the burn?
   A  First-degree burns redden the skin but do not lead to blistering.
   B  Second-degree burns include the formation of blisters as well as redness with pain.
   C  Third-degree burns affect deeper layers of the skin; they can be painless – but this means the nerves may be damaged.

## FIRST-DEGREE BURNS
## Urtica urens

◆ ordinary sunburn

*Urtica urens* is an excellent remedy to give internally for simple burns and scalds. It can also be very effective when applied externally for sunburns.

*Potency and Repetition*
For minor burns and scalds give *Urtica urens 6* every 15 minutes for five or six doses. For sunburns, soak the area with a lotion of *Urtica urens* mother tincture. This lotion should be prepared by adding 20 drops of the tincture to half a cup of cooled boiled, distilled or mineral water.

## SECOND- AND THIRD-DEGREE BURNS
## Cantharis

◆ for burns where there are **blisters**
◆ very painful burns

*Cantharis* is extremely effective where there is blistering and/or the burning is extremely painful and the child is very restless. It should be given immediately, not only in the case of second-degree but also third-degree burns, while you are waiting for additional help to arrive. It will help lessen the pain.

*Potency and Repetition*
*Cantharis 30* every 15 minutes for five or six doses.

## ALL BURNS WHERE THE SKIN IS BROKEN
## Calendula

◆ burns where **blisters have broken, with or without pus**

*Calendula* can be given internally as well as externally (see point 3 below for external use) when the blisters caused by burns have broken. This remedy is very effective in healing the skin and helping prevent infection.

*Potency and Repetition*
Give three doses of *Calendula 6* daily for three days.

### NEVER BEEN WELL SINCE A BURN
## Causticum

*Causticum* is a good remedy to give where there are areas of skin or scars that remain painful after the burns have healed.

*Potency and Repetition*
Three doses of *Causticum 30* a day for two to three days.

#### EXTERNAL AND COMMON-SENSE MEASURES
1 Remove any clothing from the burned area. If it is difficult to remove completely, cut away as much clothing as you can.
2 Apply a lotion of *Urtica urens* mother tincture (*see above, page 27*). Keep the area moist with this. Soak any clothing you have not been able to remove from the burn as well. Do not use cotton wool on open areas as it may stick to the wound.
3 When the blisters break open, apply a lotion of *Calendula* mother tincture (prepared in the same way as the *Urtica* lotion).
4 If the burn was caused by a faulty electrical appliance, unplug the unit before moving your child.
5 For chemical burns, wash with cold running water, then treat as above.
6 Do not break blisters.

#### WHEN TO SEEK PROFESSIONAL HELP
1 If the burn covers a large area of skin
2 For large second-degree burns to the hands, face, feet, ears, or genitals. Seek help also for burns to the eyes.
3 Go to the hospital or call an ambulance immediately for any third-degree burns. These burns can cause fluid loss, so get your child to drink, if at all possible, while you wait for help.
4 If your child is short of breath
5 Burns due to chemicals, acids, or caustic sodas
6 Electrical burns

## Cuts and Grazes

### Calendula

◆ **open cuts and wounds**
◆ apply **externally** as a liquid and/or ointment

*Calendula* is a wonderful healing and antiseptic agent for cuts and abrasions. All wounds should be washed first of all with *Calendula* mother tincture: put about 15 drops in half a cup of warm water. Wash the area well. Apply *Calendula* ointment, cover the wound with a plaster, leave it for two days and repeat if necessary.

*Calendula* will help the skin heal quickly and prevent any infection. If the abrasion is deep and very sensitive, some small nerve endings may have been damaged. *Hypercal* ointment, which is a combination of *Calendula* and *Hypericum,* can be very effective.

## Dental Treatment

There are some useful remedies to have at hand when your child visits the dentist. Homoeopathy can help to calm anxious patients, ease the shooting pains after fillings, and heal bruised gums.

### Aconite

◆ great **fear and panic attacks** with restlessness

*Potency and Repetition*
*Aconite 30* may be given every hour for three or four doses before the appointment.

### Arnica montana

◆ **after** any difficult **dental work**

*Arnica* is most useful when there is considerable bruising, bleeding and/or pain after any dental treatment.

*Potency and Repetition*
*Arnica 30* may be given every two hours for two or three doses, then, depending on the severity of the condition, tailed off over a day or two.

## Gelsemium

◆ **apprehension and weakness;** possible **trembling**

*Potency and Repetition*
*Gelsemium 30* may be given every two hours for two or three doses before the appointment.

## Hypericum

◆ child complains of **shooting pains** or toothache when *Arnica* has not helped
◆ **nerve damage**

*Potency and Repetition*
*Hypericum 30* may be given every two hours for up to three to four doses.

## Phosphorus

◆ **persistent bleeding** after tooth extraction

*Potency and Repetition*
*Phosphorus 30* every 15 minutes for three or four doses.

### EXTERNAL AND COMMON-SENSE MEASURES

1  If necessary, you may wash your child's mouth out with a rinse consisting of 20 drops of *Calendula* mother tincture to half a cup of cooled boiled water. This will greatly help with any bleeding and will stave off possible septic conditions. This can be done every 15 to 30 minutes.

### WHEN TO SEEK PROFESSIONAL HELP

1  If intense pain and/or bleeding persist, contact your dentist.

## Eye Injuries and Strains

The eye is a very delicate part of the body, therefore due care and attention must be given. For the purpose of this book only blows to the eyes and eye strain will be discussed.

If the vision is normal even after an injury, this is a good sign. If the vision is impaired or the pain is severe, seek help immediately. You can help your child by giving her the appropriate remedy as you wait for further treatment.

### Aconite
◆ **fear, pain and restlessness** after injury

This is the first remedy to think of when there is excessive fear and restlessness accompanied by severe pain.

*Potency and Repetition*
Give one dose of *Aconite 30* every 15 minutes for three doses. One of the following remedies may have to be given after the initial pain and fear have been reduced.

### Arnica montana
◆ black eye
◆ bloodshot eye **due to injury**

*Arnica* is the first remedy to consider for eye injuries. In cases where *Aconite* has first been given to alleviate your child's fears, *Arnica* is often the logical follow-up. It helps to reduce the pain and swelling and heal the damaged capillaries which make the eye bloodshot.

*Potency and Repetition*
*Arnica 30* every half hour for four to six doses.

If the bruising is serious and longer-term treatment is needed, give three or four doses daily for up to one week.

### Ledum
◆ **for pain, bruising, and swelling that continue after *Arnica* has been given**

*Potency and Repetition*
*Ledum 30*, two to three times a day for up to one week.

## Ruta graveolens

- **aching** of eye and eye muscles **due to over-use** or strain, e.g. reading in bad light

*Potency and Repetition*

Give one dose of *Ruta 30* every three hours for three or four doses. If this problem persists, have your child's eyes tested. If eye tests show nothing, long-term homoeopathic treatment will be needed.

## Symphytum

- **injury** to the eyeball **caused by a blunt object**
- injury to the bone around the eye

Use *Symphytum* if *Arnica* has not removed all the pain. This remedy is particularly effective if there is bruising to the bone around the eye.

*Potency and Repetition*

*Symphytum 6,* three times a day for up to one week.

### EXTERNAL AND COMMON-SENSE MEASURES

1  For all small objects lodged in the eye, such as dirt, flush the eye with a lotion made from *Euphrasia* mother tincture: 10 drops in half a cup of distilled or mineral water. If you do not have *Euphrasia,* use *Calendula* lotion made up in the same way. The common name for *Euphrasia* is Eyebright, and it is a wonderful remedy for all eye complaints.

2  For blows to the eye and the surrounding area, apply *Calendula* lotion.

### WHEN TO SEEK PROFESSIONAL HELP

1  If there is an object lodged in the eyeball. *Ledum 30* every 15 minutes may also be given while you are on the way for help.

2  Loss of, blurred or diminished vision.

3  If blood continues to collect in the eyeball or it is openly bleeding.

4  If chemicals get into the eye. Wash it out thoroughly under running tap water while you are waiting for help.

## Finger and Toe Injuries

### Hypericum

◆ **injury to nerve endings**
◆ **crushed fingertips and toes**
◆ back injuries
◆ **shooting pains**

If your child gets his fingertips caught in a door or a heavy weight falls on his toes, *Hypericum* is the first remedy to use. It helps repair the nerve endings and almost immediately relieves the pain. The skin also heals under its action. If a nail has been damaged, *Hypericum* will rapidly help it get better. If your child tumbles from a tree, or falls and injures her back (especially the tail bone), *Hypericum* will often do the trick.

*Potency and Repetition*
One dose of 30C every half hour to every three hours for three or four doses according to the intensity of the injury. If the injury seems to need longer-term treatment, one dose three or four times a day can be given over the following few days.

**EXTERNAL AND COMMON-SENSE MEASURES**
1  Alleviate bruising by placing an ice pack on the affected area. Rest and elevate the injured area.
2  *Arnica montana* can be used as an ointment, BUT MUST NEVER BE USED IN THIS WAY IF THE SKIN IS BROKEN.

**WHEN TO SEEK PROFESSIONAL HELP**
1  If the injury has been caused by something serious such as a car accident or a big fall
2  If your child loses consciousness
3  If the pain and/or numbness persist
4  If the limb will not move and you suspect a fracture
5  If there is bleeding under the skin or if the injured limb looks a bit disjointed or deformed – this may mean it has been fractured

## Fractures

A fracture is a cracked or broken bone. It is accompanied by pain and swelling. The area may possibly look deformed. Due to the intensity of the pain, and depending on the severity of the break, it may almost be impossible to move the affected limb.

### Arnica montana

◆ **first remedy** to give for initial **bruising and shock**

*Potency and Repetition*
Give one dose of *Arnica 30* every one to three hours for five or six doses. The amount of time between repeat doses can increase as your child's pain abates.

### Calcarea phosphorica

This remedy is particularly useful to give to a child who has a fracture along with a history of teething troubles or teeth which decay easily.

*Potency and Repetition*
Give one dose of *Calcarea phosphorica 6X* three times a day for up to a month to help the bone heal.

### Symphytum

◆ **broken or cracked bone**
◆ **bone refuses to heal**

*Symphytum* is the best remedy to give after *Arnica* to help heal bones. *Symphytum* by itself is a great remedy where the bone seems slow to repair itself.

*Potency and Repetition*
Give one dose of 6C three times a day for two weeks to one month, as necessary.

**EXTERNAL AND COMMON-SENSE MEASURES**

1 If you suspect your child has a fracture, do not move the injured part.
2 Undiluted *Symphytum* mother tincture can be dabbed on the area with cotton wool, especially if the fracture is close to the surface.
3 Gently clean any area that is exposed and bleeding while you are waiting for help (*see* **Cuts and Grazes**, *page 29*). If the bleeding is severe, you may have to apply pressure to stop it.

**WHEN TO SEEK PROFESSIONAL HELP**

An X-ray is usually necessary to diagnose a fracture.

1 If you suspect your child has sustained a fracture.
2 If the injured part is distorted or deformed.
3 If there is bleeding under the skin (may suggest a fracture).
4 If the injury is very painful and your child cannot move it.
5 If pain continues for some days in the injured part (the bone may have cracked).

## Head Injuries

### Arnica montana

◆ **at the beginning, first remedy to consider**
◆ no other indications

*Arnica*, here as elsewhere, is one of the first remedies to consider. It will help with bleeding, bruises, pain and shock. In most simple cases it is all that will be needed.

*Potency and Repetition*

One dose of 30C every half hour to every three hours for five or six doses.

## Hypericum

♦ **damage to the nerves in the neck after a head injury**

*Hypericum* is a useful remedy for whiplash or any other injury to the nerves in the neck. It is especially indicated if pains start shooting down the arm.

### Potency and Repetition
One dose of 12C twice daily for up to three weeks.

## Natrum sulphuricum

♦ pains **that continue after head injuries**
♦ mental or emotional changes that continue after an injury
♦ **never been well since a head injury**

*Natrum sulphuricum* is often considered after a head injury has not responded completely to *Arnica*. It is also indicated where there are some changes in the child's personality, for the worse.

### Potency and Repetition
Three doses of *Natrum sulphuricum 200* One dose in the morning, one dose the same evening, and one dose the following morning.

### EXTERNAL AND COMMON-SENSE MEASURES
1  Clean any wounds and/or bleeding as suggested in the **Cuts and Grazes** section.

### WHEN TO SEEK PROFESSIONAL HELP
Children are often banging and bumping their heads; in most cases these injuries present no real problem. If severe, however, they can lead to very serious consequences, which may not be obvious in the beginning. You should go to the hospital or call an ambulance immediately if the following are present:

1  Any loss or change in consciousness within the first 48 hours after the bang or fall
2  Injury caused by a very heavy object, a major fall or serious accident
3  Bleeding or loss of fluid from the nose or ear

4  Increased sleepiness or drowsiness
5  Any signs of damage to the nervous system, such as blurred or double vision, slurred speech, weakness in the arms or legs, convulsions, different size of pupils or unusual eye movements
6  Unusual irritability, confusion, or restlessness
7  Vomiting
8  Neck pain or tenderness

## Insect Bites and Stings

### Apis mellifica

◆ **heat, redness and swelling**
◆ **relieved by cool applications**

*Apis* naturally follows *Ledum* (see below) for insect bites. The area swells rapidly and is painful, burning or itching.

*Potency and Repetition*
One dose every 15 to 30 minutes for three to five doses.

### Ledum

◆ **the first remedy for stings**
◆ mosquito bites
◆ bee or wasp stings, etc.

Stings are in a sense a type of puncture wound, and *Ledum* is very useful for these types of wounds.

*Potency and Repetition*
One dose of *Ledum 30* every half hour for three to four doses.

As a prophylactic for children sensitive to mosquito bites, *Ledum 30* can be given three times on the day before going to an infested area. Three more doses can be given on the day of arrival. If this seems to help, further occasional doses as needed can be given. Use *Ledum* in this way only for acute treatment. For more permanent results, you should seek out constitutional homoeopathic treatment.

## Urtica urens

◆ **itching and stinging (as with hives or nettle rash)**

*Potency and Repetition*

One dose of *Urtica urens 30C* every 15 to 60 minutes for four or five doses, as necessary.

**EXTERNAL AND COMMON-SENSE MEASURES**

1  Use mosquito repellent.
2  In the case of stings, try to remove the stinger with tweezers.
3  Dab the area with *Ledum* undiluted mother tincture.
4  If extreme itching persists, apply undiluted *Urtica urens* mother tincture to the area.
5  A slice of onion applied to the sting may help relieve the pain.

**WHEN TO SEEK PROFESSIONAL HELP**

1  If your child is known to react very badly to stings
2  If breathing becomes difficult
3  If the bite is from something known to be extremely poisonous

## Nosebleeds

Nosebleeds are a frequent problem in children. The following remedies are for simple nosebleeds caused by injury, not for recurrent nosebleeds. Trauma to the nose includes blows, nose-picking and sticking foreign bodies up the nose. Nosebleeds can also be associated with coughs and/or fevers. See the relevant sections for this. If the problem is a chronic, recurrent one, seek professional homoeopathic help.

## Aconite

◆ **great fear and anxiety with bleeding**

*Potency and Repetition*

One dose every 10 to 15 minutes for three or four doses. The first dose may alleviate your child's fear; if the bleeding persists, follow this treatment with one of the following:

## Arnica montana

◆ nosebleed after **blows, injuries**

*Potency and Repetition*
One dose of *Arnica 30* every 10 to 15 minutes for three to four doses.

## Phosphorus

◆ **if *Arnica* fails**
◆ bleeding caused by violent blowing of the nose

*Potency and Repetition*
One dose of *Phosphorus 30* every 15 to 30 minutes (depending on the severity of the bleeding) for three or four doses.

**EXTERNAL AND COMMON-SENSE MEASURES**

1  Pinch the soft part of the nose (just below the bony part) for 10 minutes. As you do this, have your child lean forward over a table. If the bleeding persists, repeat.
2  Make sure there is nothing up your child's nose. If there is, remove it yourself or seek help in getting it removed.
3  An ice pack may help stop the bleeding.
4  Make sure your child doesn't lie in a position that will allow her to swallow the blood.
5  A tissue soaked in *Hamamelis* (witch hazel) mother tincture and inserted in the nose may help stop the bleeding.

**WHEN TO SEEK PROFESSIONAL HELP**

1  If profuse bleeding persists
2  If there is any other bruising accompanying the nosebleed – for example if your child has had a fall; recurrent nosebleeds can be a sign of concussion

## Puncture Wounds

*see* **Animal Bites and Puncture Wounds**

## Shock

### Aconite

◆ **after-effects of a fright,** severe **shock**
◆ loss of blood, especially when accompanied by **fright**
◆ extreme fears, especially **fear of death**

*Aconite* is often indicated for injuries where the child is extremely fearful and restless, or if she is bleeding and her fright becomes overwhelming. This remedy will help calm the child down; other remedies can be given for the specific physical problem as needed.

*Aconite* is generally most useful when a problem begins. See the specific physical problem for remedies that may be used after *Aconite.*

*Potency and Repetition*
*Aconite 30* should be given immediately. It can be given every 15 to 30 minutes for three doses, or until your child calms down. If this is the correct remedy your child will usually relax within half an hour; she may even go to sleep.

## Sprains and Strains

These are caused by the sudden tearing of tissues and muscles. A sprain is an injury around a joint and is usually accompanied by tenderness with pain and swelling. A strain happens to a muscle and is accompanied by sudden sharp pains and swelling.

### Arnica montana

◆ **first remedy** to give
◆ **bruising, pain and swelling**
◆ shock from injury

*Arnica* is the first remedy to think of for either sprains or strains – or indeed for any injury. It will help deal with any initial shock and bruising. For best results, follow up your use of *Arnica* with one of the remedies listed below.

*Potency and Repetition*
One dose of *Arnica 6* should be given anywhere from every half hour to every three hours for three to five doses according to the severity of the pain and swelling.

## Bryonia

♦ joint or muscle pains
♦ **sharp pains**
♦ hot, swollen joints
♦ **pains that are made worse by even the slightest movement**

*Bryonia* can be useful for muscles that are injured and are accompanied by sharp, stitching pains. These pains will be sharper if there is any motion at all, even a motion as slight as breathing.

*Potency and Repetition*
One dose of *Bryonia 30* every three to four hours for two to three days, as necessary.

## Rhus toxicodendron

♦ sprained **joints**
♦ pulled muscles, **swollen joints from injury**

This type of pain will feel worse when the child first starts to move the affected area, but will lessen as the motion continues.

*Rhus toxicodendron* is one of the primary remedies in homoeopathic medicine for these injuries accompanied by swelling, stiffness and bruised pain, and often follows *Arnica* well. Frequently the pain will decrease as gentle motion continues. If you observe this in your child, *Rhus toxicodendron* is definitely the remedy to give. *Rhus toxicodendron*, however, will often help after *Arnica* even if the pain is not made better by movement.

*Potency and Repetition*
*Rhus toxicodendron 30* every hour to every three hours for the first day. After that give it three times a day for two to three days more.

## Ruta graveolens

◆ **damage to cartilage of bones and tendons**
◆ injuries **where the bones are close to surface** (in those cases where it might be easy for the bone to be damaged)

*Ruta graveolens* is another remedy that follows *Arnica* well in injuries where there is bruised aching, the bones are injured, and/or tendons have been overstretched. If *Rhus toxicodendron* or *Bryonia* have not effected a cure, this remedy will help. It can be especially useful for injuries around the wrists and ankles.

*Potency and Repetition*
One dose of *Ruta 6C* three times a day for up to three weeks as necessary.

## Strontium carbonicum

◆ lingering **ankle sprain**
◆ repeated ankle sprains

*Strontium carbonicum* should be considered where there is a swollen, sprained ankle that has not responded well to other remedies. It can also be considered as a first-aid remedy for recurrent ankle sprains.

*Potency and Repetition*
One dose of 6C three times a day for up to three weeks.

**EXTERNAL AND COMMON-SENSE MEASURES**
1  There is a formula called RICE that is always helpful:
   **R** = Rest. Make sure your child and her injured limb get enough rest.
   **I** = Ice. Apply an ice pack to the injured area.
   **C** = Compression. Wrap a tight bandage around the injured part.
   **E** = Elevation. Keep the injured part elevated.
2  *Arnica* may also be applied as an ointment, as long as there is no broken skin.
3  If there is an open wound and/or bleeding, clean the wound with the measures listed in the **Cuts and Grazes** section, and take steps to stop the bleeding.

**WHEN TO SEEK PROFESSIONAL HELP**

1  If the pain of a strain persists or is very intense, and the injured area is impossible to move
2  If an affected limb looks shortened, distorted, blue, numb or cold

Administering the appropriate remedy on the way to the doctor or hospital will help immensely.

## Stings

*see* **Insect Bites and Stings**

## Sun Stroke and Heat Sickness

Sunstroke can be a serious problem. The temperature regulation mechanism may temporarily stop functioning properly. Along with making her feel hot, dry and red, this can make your child confused, weak, dizzy and faint. She may also experience muscle cramps, and have difficulty breathing. If the symptoms seem serious, do not hesitate to seek help.

### Belladonna

◆ **face is very red and hot**
◆ **throbbing headache**
◆ sensitivity to light

*Belladonna* is a remedy to consider when the symptoms come on quickly. This remedy presents a picture of great intensity – of heat, redness and dryness. Your child's face and eyes will be extremely red and hot. She will be highly agitated and may have a severe, pounding headache.

*Potency and Repetition*
One dose of *Belladonna 30* every 15 minutes for five or six doses.

## Cuprum metallicum

◆ severe **muscular cramping or twitching** along with possible sweats after exposure to sun

*Potency and Repetition*
One dose of *Cuprum 30* every half hour.

## Glonoine

◆ blood rushes to the head
◆ **sense of head bursting**
◆ mental confusion

*Glonoine* is similar to *Belladonna*. The blood rushes into the head and may produce confusion. Your child's face will be red and she may experience a sensation that her head is expanding or will burst. If there is no improvement after two or three doses of *Belladonna*, try *Glonoine* (or vice versa).

*Potency and Repetition*
One dose of *Glonoine 30* every 15 minutes for five or six doses.

## Natrum carbonicum

◆ **weakness** from exposure to the sun
◆ **nausea** and/or diarrhoea from exposure to the sun

*Natrum carbonicum* does not usually show the same intensity as *Belladonna* and is usually indicated for problems brought on by heat exhaustion, rather than for severe heat stroke. Your child will feel very, very weak and possibly dizzy. She may also feel nauseated and/or have diarrhoea.

*Potency and Repetition*
One dose of *Natrum carbonicum 30* every half hour.

**EXTERNAL AND COMMON-SENSE MEASURES**

1  For the first few days of summer or when on holiday in a hot climate, take care. Make sure that your child does not stay out in the open sun all day. Keep her covered up with sunblock and a hat. These simple precautions are easy to forget but can save your child a lot of discomfort.

2 If your child gets a sunburn, treat as directed on page 26
   (**Burns and Scalds**).
3 If the heat stroke or exhaustion is severe, drinking a solution
   of a quarter to a half teaspoon of salt in half a litre of water
   every half hour can help with dehydration.
4 Place a cold compress on your child's head; cool her body
   down with wet cloths.

**WHEN TO SEEK PROFESSIONAL HELP**

1 True sunstroke requires immediate medical attention. If your
   child's body temperature rises very rapidly this can quickly
   lead to collapse. This can damage important organs of the
   body. If this happens, give *Belladonna* or *Glonoine* while
   waiting for help.

## Toe Injuries

*see* **Finger and Toe Injuries**

chapter five

# homoeopathic treatment for everyday complaints

## Bedwetting

Bedwetting (enuresis) can simply be the result of a delay in the maturity of the part of the brain that controls urination, so try not to make too much of a fuss about it. It is only considered to be a 'problem' if your child is over six. If you are worried, check with your doctor to be sure there is nothing wrong with your child's bladder, and then seek homoeopathic help.

Sometimes bedwetting may be a sign that your child for some reason wants attention during the night. Perhaps he has not seen enough of you during the day. If no other cause can be found, it may be an emotional issue that is at the heart of the problem. Even teenagers have been known to wet the bed during stressful times. And numerous other theories abound: jealousy at the birth of a new sibling, a change of residence, problems at school, family stresses such as grief or fear. A child may simply be of a rather nervous disposition, or perhaps he was toilet trained before he was truly physically ready. Very occasionally there is a physical problem, such as cystitis. For this you will need professional help. In some instances where no cause seems apparent, constitutional treatment may be necessary.

## Causticum

◆ **child wets the bed in the first part of the night**, soon after falling asleep
◆ **may involuntarily lose urine during the day** if overexcited, coughing or sneezing

## Equisetum

◆ **if your child has no symptoms and common-sense measures have not helped**
◆ child has dreams of urinating
◆ if other remedies have not helped

## Kreosote

◆ for sound **sleepers** who are **difficult to wake up**
◆ **child dreams of urinating**, often while wetting the bed

## Pulsatilla

◆ **timid, sweet, weepy, affectionate children**
◆ clingy to parents
◆ prefer open air; dislike heat

## Sepia

◆ **wets the bed in the first part of sleep**
◆ **more commonly used with girls**
◆ child likes sports, dancing or rapid movement
◆ usually prefers to be alone

### *Potency and Repetition*

One dose of 30C of the appropriate remedy every 12 hours for three doses; then wait for two weeks. If the remedy helps at first but then there is a relapse, repeat the course of treatment one more time. If there is another relapse, seek the help of a qualified homoeopath.

**EXTERNAL AND COMMON-SENSE MEASURES**

1 Make sure your child goes to the toilet last thing before bed.
2 Limit his fluid intake during the evening.
3 Lift him from bed and take him to the toilet before you go to sleep.
4 Go to your doctor or homoeopath to check for urinary infections.

5  If the bedwetting starts suddenly when there have been no previous problems, check for allergies and food sensitivities (has a new food been introduced into your child's diet?).

6  Do not scold or shame your child. He will already be feeling demoralized, even if he does not show it. Try to work together in a positive way to overcome the difficulties.

7  Limit his intake of salty and spicy foods (which could lead him to drink more).

8  Try to make sure the lower parts of your child's body are covered up and warm at night.

9  Some studies have shown that watching a violent or disturbing television programme before bed can lead to bedwetting.

## Circumcision

One dose of *Arnica 200* about one hour before the circumcision, and a second dose as quickly afterwards as possible. About one hour after the second dose of *Arnica*, give one dose of *Staphysagria 30*.

These remedies will help ease the pain for a child of any age, as well as promote quick healing.

*Staphysagria* helps with urinary difficulties and, in older children, will ease any feelings of humiliation caused by the need to have a circumcision.

## Colds, Coughs and Chest Complaints

These conditions, as well as sore throats (which are given their own section – *see pages 111–115*),are often hard to distinguish one from the other, as their symptoms can be very similar and most children seem to run from one complaint into another. There are many different remedies available for the variations that can appear, and they cannot all be covered in a book such as this. We have provided the most commonly indicated remedies here, and have divided the complaints into two main groups to try to make it easier for you to pick the right remedy. You may also want to consult the other relevant sections in this book.

### BRONCHITIS

This generally starts as a cold with fever, malaise and a sore throat, followed by a cough. The cough is often dry and painful to begin with, later producing phlegm. There may be wheezing or whistling sounds during breathing.

Bronchitis is common in children and can happen after exposure to cold, damp or dry weather. It can also take place during teething and can linger for two to three weeks. Bronchitis can become chronic. Some children seem to have a predisposition to bronchitis. *Chronic cases need constitutional treatment* by a professional homoeopath.

## Aconite, Belladonna and Ferrum phosphoricum

May be indicated in the beginning. *See* the **Colds**, **Cough** and **Croup** sections for indications, potency and dosage.

## Antimonium tartaricum

- ◆ **rattling of mucus in the chest**
- ◆ child is extremely **drowsy**
- ◆ may want to sit up
- ◆ **child is pale and sweaty, or may be blue around the lips**

*Antimonium tartaricum* is useful in the late stages of bronchitis. Compare with *Ipecacuanha*, below.

When *Antimonium tartaricum* is usually indicated your child is very ill. As well as giving him this remedy, you should seek the help of a doctor or professional homoeopath.

## Bryonia

- ◆ **dry cough** which may hurt your child's head and chest
- ◆ dry mouth with **thirst for large quantities of water**
- ◆ aversion to being too warm
- ◆ **worse from moving,** prefers to lie still
- ◆ **dryness** of mouth and lips; constipation

## Dulcamara

- **during a sudden change in the weather (from warm to cold)**
- **during times when the days are warm and the nights cold**
- child produces a lot of mucus
- increased urination

## Hepar sulphuris

- **child is very chilly and feels worse for all things cold**
- **extremely oversensitive to all things**, such as touch, pain, cold air, cold draughts
- **prefers warm drinks**
- may have splinter-like sensations in chest
- **sweats at night**
- may be irritable

## Ipecacuanha

- spasmodic **coughing with** possible **nausea and/or vomiting**
- chest full of **rattling mucus**
- the child is **too weak to bring up mucus**
- **wheezing**
- clean, **pink tongue**
- **worse for** motion and **open air**
- nose bleeds caused by the coughing

*Ipecacuanha* is usually indicated at the beginning of a bronchitis that comes on very rapidly. *Antimonium tartaricum* is indicated later on. *Ipecacuanha* is commonly used where there is a combination of wheezing along with nausea and/or retching.

## Kali carbonicum

- **worse early morning** (between 2 and 5 a.m.)
- **worse for cold air**
- child **needs to sit up** or lean forward

## Mercurius vivus

- excessive **perspiration at night**
- **increased salivation** – may dribble on pillow
- **bad breath**
- mucus coughed up from chest

### Phosphorus

◆ **thirst for cold drinks**
◆ **wheezing and coughing worse for talking and laughing**
◆ very **tight, constricted chest** as if a weight is on it
◆ **anxious,** fearful, **needs company**

### Pulsatilla

◆ **dry cough at night which often forces the child to sit up**
◆ cough is **worse in a warm room; child wants open air**
◆ **little or no thirst, even if feverish**
◆ may take a sip of drink only because his mouth is dry, not because he feels thirsty
◆ weepy, with a **desire for company**

*Potency and Repetition*

One dose of 12 or 30C of the appropriate remedy every three to five hours for two or three days. The frequency of repetition depends on the intensity of the bronchitis. Lengthen the amount of time between doses as your child starts to improve.

#### COLDS

Common colds affect all of us. They account for more time off school than any other cause. Many treatments are offered at the chemist for colds, but none is curative; they only help give temporary relief to the symptoms. Homoeopaths believe that colds should be allowed to run their course. Discharges are the body's way of expelling toxins and should not be suppressed. Only if a cold is severe is homoeopathic treatment really necessary to aid the body's natural recovery process.

The symptoms vary in intensity but generally start with a runny nose, malaise, sneezing and often a sore throat and coughing. As a cold progresses the 'stuffed up feeling' passes and the runny nose and discharge may become thickened and possibly green or yellow. In some children a cold may develop into a chest complaint or be associated with ear problems.

Some children seem to get repeated colds or to have constant colds with runny noses. These children should be treated constitutionally.

## Aconite

- at the beginning
- **sudden, intense onset**
- after **exposure to dry, cold wind**
- extreme **restlessness, anxiety and fear**
- **high fever**
- **chest** may be affected and **croup** is common
- rapid, hard pulse
- choking cough

## Belladonna

- at the beginning
- **sudden, intense onset**
- **flushed, hot, bright red face**
- **high fever**
- **sensitivity to light**
- **hot head with cold feet** and hands
- often affects the **throat or glands**
- delirium

## Ferrum phosphoricum

- **at the beginning of colds with fever and no other symptoms**
- flushed cheeks

## Gelsemium

- often worse for warm, moist weather
- slow onset
- low-grade fever
- **heaviness, weakness, tiredness, dizziness**
- **child keeps still**; wants no one around
- **drooping eyelids** – child can hardly keep them open
- no thirst
- aching limbs and back
- slow, weak pulse

The above four remedies are usually more useful at the beginning of colds or inflammations. *Aconite* and *Belladonna* are best for a cold that comes on rapidly and is very intense at the outset. *Gelsemium* is for colds that develop more slowly; the symptoms of *Ferrum phosphoricum* arise at a pace somewhere between the two.

*Potency and Repetition*

Choose the correct remedy according to the symptoms. Give one dose of 12C or 30C according to the intensity of the symptoms every 15 minutes, half hour or hour, for a few doses. You will probably have to repeat the dosage of *Belladonna* or *Aconite* quite frequently. Gelsemium can usually be repeated every three to four hours.

## Allium cepa

- **eyes and nose** run
- **burning discharge from nose, making the upper lip red and sore**
- **child feels better in the open air**
- tickling in the larynx
- non-irritating discharge from the eyes

## Arsenicum album

- **nasal discharge which reddens the skin**
- burning in nose
- child feels **chilly; is better near heat**
- **restless**, anxious, fearful

## Dulcamara

- after **exposure to cold, wet weather**
- child gets **chilled or wet after being warm or overheated**

## Euphrasia

- opposite of *Allium cepa*
- **running eyes and burning discharge from the eyes and bland, non-irritating discharge from the nose**
- **cough is worse during the daytime**

## Kali bichromicum

- **thick yellow, ropey discharge difficult to expel**

## Nux vomica

- irritability
- child **desires warmth**
- **the slightest movement increases the chill**

## Pulsatilla

◆ child is **clingy, weepy**
◆ does not want to be alone
◆ usually no thirst
◆ **likes open air**
◆ **thick yellow-green mucus**

## Rhus toxicodendron

◆ child is **restless**, can't keep still
◆ **worse for cold, damp weather**
◆ **tosses and turns in bed**

## Sticta

◆ needs **to blow nose but nothing comes out**
◆ **dryness with obstruction and pressure, especially at root of nose**

*Potency and Repetition*

One dose of 12 or 30C every three hours for three to five doses. Stop the remedy when your child is definitely getting better.

### COUGHS AND CHEST COMPLAINTS

Coughs are often protective in that they serve to expel mucus from the respiratory tract. They can be shallow or deep, dry or productive. Noticing these differences will help you to choose a remedy.

Generally, as with colds, homoeopaths prefer not to treat coughs unless they are prolonged, very distressing, or there seems to be a danger of a more serious disorder developing.

*The treatment of coughs can sometimes be difficult. Distinguishing characteristic symptoms requires careful observation.*

We have broken the chest complaints into specific types. There is also a section here on *coughs in general.* You will often find that the symptoms (and remedies) seem to overlap, so you may have to look from section to section to find the most suitable remedy.

If coughs continue or have a tendency to return, consult a professional homoeopath about constitutional treatment.

### COUGHS (IN GENERAL)

Can be caused by a simple inflammation, often after exposure to sudden or extreme weather conditions. They may also be due to allergies. Coughs can accompany a simple cold or can progress to bronchitis, pneumonia or asthma. Children may have a constitutional tendency to repeated coughs and you should ask a professional homoeopath for assistance. Refer to **Bronchitis** and **Colds** for more indications and remedies that may not be listed in this section.

At the outset:

### Aconite
◆ **dry, sudden cough after exposure to dry, cold wind**

*See* **Colds** and **Croup** for more indications.

### Belladonna
◆ child is **extremely hot, with a flushed red face**

*See* **Colds** and **Croup** for more indications.

### Ferrum phosphoricum
◆ **short, tickling cough, with few other symptoms**

*See* **Colds** for more indications.

*Potency and Repetition*
One dose of 12 or 30C every one to two hours, depending on the intensity of the symptoms, for three doses. If three doses do not provide relief, you have not chosen the correct remedy. If one of the above remedies has helped but then seems to stop working, the picture may have changed and another remedy may be needed.

### Antimonium tartaricum
*See* **Bronchitis**

## Bryonia

- **a hard dry cough** which may hurt the chest
- **thirst for cool drinks**
- **worse for motion**
- child **prefers to be alone,** may be irritable
- cough or chest pain is **worse when breathing deeply**
- child may hold his hand to his chest – he finds this helps to keep him from moving
- may have a headache from coughing so much

## Drosera

*See* **Croup** and **Whooping Cough**

## Hepar sulphuris

*See* **Bronchitis**

## Ipecacuanha

*See* **Bronchitis**

## Kali bichromicum

- **thick, tough, ropey yellowish mucus from chest and/or nose that is difficult to bring up**
- hacking cough with a tickle in the pit of the throat

## Manganum

- cough **is better when lying down** and resting; **often occurs only during the day**
- **worse in cold, damp weather**

## Phosphorus

- **thirst for cool drinks or fruit juice**
- may have a headache from coughing
- **cough is worse for talking, laughing, cool air**
- child needs company
- **fear of the dark**
- child feels **chilly**
- worse when lying on the left side

## Pulsatilla

- **dry cough during the evening**
- cough may be loose in the morning
- thick, yellow mucus
- **worse in a warm room, prefers open air**
- child is **mild**, affectionate, **wants company**
- **cough is better for sitting up**

## Rhus toxicodendron

- **restlessness** – needs to move
- **cough may be better for motion**
- coughs during sleep
- **worse for exposure to cold damp** – even exposing an arm out of his blanket aggravates the cough

## Rumex

- cough **due to tickling in the throat or chest**
- **worse** in cold air, especially when **inhaling cold air**

## Spongia

- **dry, harsh, hoarse cough**
- prefers warm drinks
- **wakes from sleep feeling suffocated** because of the cough
- **cough may sound like a saw going through wood**

*Potency and Repetition*

One dose of 12 or 30C every four hours for four to six doses. Stop, or increase the length of time between doses, as your child begins to improve.

### CROUP

This is the name given to a hoarse, metallic-sounding cough usually centred around the larynx (voice box). It often causes the child to wake up at night, though he can seem better during the day.

Children from three months to four years old are often susceptible to croup. The cough can last as long as three to four days and be very distressing to watch. Its duration and intensity can be helped greatly by homoeopathic remedies.

### Aconite

- child **wakes in the night with dry, hoarse, barking cough, restless and anxious**
- **one of the first remedies for sudden croup, especially if it starts at night**

*See* **Colds** for more indications.

### Belladonna

- **high fever with flushed red face and dry, barking, painful cough**

*See* **Colds** for more indications.

### Ferrum phosphoricum

*See* **Colds** for indications.

*Potency and Repetition*

The three above remedies may be given in either 12C or 30C; one dose every half hour for two to three doses will usually be enough. This will either clear up the condition completely or at least let you and your child sleep. If the symptoms do not clear up, another remedy may be indicated – try one of the following.

### Drosera

- **dry, barking or ringing metallic-sounding cough**
- **cough worse when lying down** or as soon as the child's head hits his pillow
- cough may come from deep in chest
- cough **may end in vomiting**
- **worse for** eating or **drinking**

## Hepar sulphuris

◆ often follows *Spongia* well (see below)
◆ **useful in the later stages** of croup, rarely the beginning
◆ usually the mucus **rattles** more than if *Spongia* or *Aconite* is required – cough is much looser
◆ worse early in the morning
◆ **worse for all things cold** – food, air, drinks
◆ **chilly**, needs warmth
◆ coughs or sneezes when exposed to cold things

## Spongia

◆ follows *Aconite* well (see above)
◆ **dry, hard, harsh, hoarse, ringing-sounding cough**
◆ cough sounds **like a saw going through dry wood**
◆ loud**, barking cough**
◆ sometimes child **wakes** with a cough just **before or around midnight**
◆ sense of **suffocation** due to **constriction of the throat or larynx**
◆ better for warm drinks
◆ **worse** when the child inhales, **talks**, sings or swallows

*Potency and Repetition*

One dose of 12 or 30C every two to three hours for three to five doses. Stop when your child shows signs of improvement.

### LARYNGITIS

An inflammation of the voice box. It is usually associated with colds, whooping cough or measles. Other causes can be excessive mouth-breathing, allergies and/or pollutants. The signs of laryngitis are hoarseness or even a complete loss of the voice. Your child may complain of pain when speaking and/or swallowing. May be accompanied by a dry cough. Generally laryngitis resolves itself, though some children have a tendency to recurrent laryngitis and need constitutional care.

At the outset:

## Aconite

*See* **Colds, Coughs** and **Croup**

## Belladonna

*See* **Colds, Coughs** and **Croup**

## Ferrum phosphoricum

◆ **at the outset, when there are no clear symptoms**
◆ there may be a nosebleed

*Potency and Repetition*

One dose of 12 or 30C every half hour to every two hours, depending on the intensity of the symptoms, for three or four doses.

## Causticum

◆ **after exposure to cold weather or dry, cold wind**
◆ a **sense of rawness** may be present
◆ hoarseness that is **worse in the morning**
◆ child may leak urine while coughing

## Phosphorus

◆ hoarseness is **worse in the evening**
◆ child is **thirsty for cool drinks**
◆ there may be a hard, painful cough

## Rumex

◆ tickling in the larynx, **worse for inhaling cool air**

## Spongia

◆ **dry, burning, tight sensation** in larynx
◆ **larynx sensitive to touch**

*See* **Croup** for more indications

*Potency and Repetition*

One dose of 12 or 30C three times a day for two or three days. Discontinue the remedy when your child gets better. If there is a relapse, repeat the remedy one or two more times at three-hourly intervals.

**EXTERNAL AND COMMON-SENSE MEASURES**

1  Try to stop your child from talking, to give his voice a rest.
2  Give him lots of warm fluids, such as honey and lemon drinks.
3  Steam inhalation will help, as will a humidifier kept going in the sick room.

### PNEUMONIA

An inflammation of the lung tissue itself. Your child may have a fever up to 40.5°C (105°F); in some cases there may be convulsions. Your child will sweat, his breathing will be rapid and he will look absolutely wretched. His sputum may be blood-streaked and he may feel nauseated or vomit. *If you suspect pneumonia at all or are the least bit uncertain, seek help immediately.* This can be a serious condition which you should not try to treat yourself. You can give the indicated remedy from the **Bronchitis** section while you are waiting for additional help.

#### EXTERNAL AND COMMON-SENSE MEASURES

1  Be alert to your child's breathing.
2  Holding and rocking your child can relax and comfort him.
3  Give him fluids: water and fruit juices (warm).
4  Steam inhalations or a humidifier will help.
5  If you have no steam inhaler or humidifier, turn on the hot water in the bathroom, fill it with steam and have your child sit in there for about a half hour. This heat will not help every child so check on how he feels after the first 10 minutes or so.
6  Be patient.
7  Make sure your child gets plenty of rest.
8  *Also see* **Fevers**
9  Give your child 1 gram of vitamin C per day.
10  For coughs and colds, cut up a large red onion, boil it in a pint of water, add a pinch of salt and a pat of butter, simmer until the onion is soft and give it to your child to drink (as hot as he can stand). This helps stimulate perspiration.
11  Wash 2 oz/50 g of barley and boil it in 1 pint/500 ml of water for about 10 minutes. Discard the water. Recook in 4 pints/2 litres of water, boiling it down to 2 pints/1 litre. Strain, add honey and feed this water to your child. This is often useful for colds.

12  Grate a piece of ginger the size of the top half of your thumb
    and boil in 1½ pints/750 ml of water for 20 minutes. Add
    honey to each cupful you give your child. This is very
    helpful for colds and chest congestion, and can be given
    several times during the day. You can dilute this ginger drink
    with more water if it is too strong for your child.
13  Avoid feeding your child dairy products, raw foods, sweet
    drinks or sweets, as these may encourage mucus production.

### WHEN TO SEEK PROFESSIONAL HELP

1   If your child's breathing is shallow and rapid
2   If your child stops breathing for a moment
3   If he is blue in the face, lips or nails; if his limbs feel cold
4   If he has a persistent high fever, with or without shallow
    breathing
5   Go to the hospital if your child inhales anything that cannot
    be coughed up and/or causes violent coughing
6   If there is any change in consciousness: drowsiness, confusion,
    convulsions
7   If your child coughs up blood
8   If he complains of chest pain
9   If he vomits along with coughing
10  If the cough or cold has not improved after a week to 10 days

## Case Study

With children so many crises seem to occur at night or at the
weekend. Ear infections, coughs and fevers often begin with a
screaming cry in the middle of the night. A familiar scene is an
anxious mother trying to describe the symptoms to a very sleepy
homoeopath over the phone at 2 a.m.

Peter, eight, woke up at three in the morning with a very severe
cough. It was a 'croupy type' cough. He became very distressed and
unable to breathe. His face began to turn red. He was unable to catch
his breath between coughs. His mother wisely took him into the
bathroom, turned on the shower to steam up the room, opened the
window, then ran to the phone. The child was extremely fearful. In

between coughs he would say in a choking voice that he was going to die. His mother described him as looking fearful and anxious, his eyes wide, pupils dilated and his face bright red. The cough sounded very dry, like the barking of a seal. Peter did not want to be held and consoled. He was frightened, yet did not really want reassurance.

He refused anything to drink to help stop the cough. The previous day he had been fine and happy, playing football in the afternoon – his mother said she could not believe his stamina. It had started to rain while the football game was going on, but that had not deterred him. He played even harder in the second half.

With this last bit of information the pieces of the puzzle that make up a remedy 'picture' fell into place. The suddenness of the onset, the fearful look in his eyes, the sound of the cough, the redness of the face. We recommended *Aconite 200* (luckily Peter's mum had some in the house). The next day she called to say that, within five minutes, Peter had settled down. In 15 minutes he was back in bed and slept through the night quietly. In the morning he was fine.

The correctly indicated homoeopathic remedy can act so quickly it seems like a miracle.

## Convulsions

A seizure or convulsion is a brief disorder of the brain accompanied by a change in consciousness, and twitching and/or jerking of the limbs. There may be breathing difficulties, rolling of the eyes, leakage of urine or stools. The seizure may last some seconds or even minutes. It is sometimes accompanied by a high fever and is very frightening for parents to witness.

Fits may also happen during teething, with whooping cough, after emotional upsets, or independently of any obvious cause. If the fits happen along with another problem, refer to the relevant section of this book as well.

*If your child is having a convulsion for any reason at all, stay with him, place him on his side and have someone call an ambulance immediately.* While you are waiting for help, if the fit is accompanied by a high fever you can sponge your child down with tepid water and try the following remedies.

## Belladonna

- ◆ **seizures with high fever, burning skin, wild staring eyes and a flushed face**
- ◆ twitching, jerking, trembling
- ◆ **comes on suddenly**
- ◆ throbbing fontanelle (infants only)

## Chamomilla

- ◆ **convulsions that occur during teething**
- ◆ child is very upset and irritable
- ◆ **worse at night**, from 9 p.m. on
- ◆ one cheek red, the other pale
- ◆ convulsions **caused by anger**
- ◆ green, loose stools

## Cuprum metallicum

- ◆ **convulsions that accompany whooping cough**

*Potency and Repetition*

One dose of 12 or 30C immediately. If one dose helps, leave it. If the fits continue or keep recurring, give the remedy every 15 minutes, or at the time of the relapse, until help arrives.

## Digestive Problems

Digestive tract illnesses such as vomiting, nausea, colic, diarrhoea and constipation are quite common in children. Usually they present no real problem and, depending on their severity, can be managed. Frequently the symptoms of one problem can 'overlap' with another, so you may have to refer to the different sub-sections below in order to find the most suitable remedy.

Most of the complications and situations that may indicate a need for professional help are listed at the end of this section (*see page 74*).

### APPENDICITIS

This is rare in young children, but very difficult to diagnose. Vomiting may be the major sign in a very young child. In older children it is abdominal tenderness centred over the right lower abdomen. The pain is often worse when your child moves. Appendicitis is most often indicated by two additional factors.

1 **Guarding**:
*a stiffening of the muscles in the sore area when approached*
2 **Rebound Tenderness**:
the area is not painful when pressed, but does hurt when the pressure is eased

Professional help should always be sought if you suspect your child has appendicitis. If the pain in the area is severe, go to the hospital immediately.

## Bryonia

◆ this remedy fits the two above symptoms well. It is one of the best remedies to consider while you are awaiting help.

*Potency and Repetition*
Give one dose of 30C every 15 to 30 minutes until you receive help or there is significant improvement.

## Iris tenax

6C every 15 to 30 minutes for a few doses while waiting for or seeking help – this has been found helpful in some cases where symptoms are not marked.

### COLIC

This is a name for severe abdominal pain which comes and goes with variable intensity. Infantile colic can begin a few days after birth and can last up to three months. It is caused in babies and young children by spasmodic contractions of the intestines and distension caused by gas. Colic occurs because the digestive tract is still maturing.

Your child may have a normal appetite and be gaining weight, yet may still howl with pain after meals. Colic is a common problem, yet there is no known reason why it happens to some children and not others.

Infantile colic can be extremely distressing for parents and their child alike. It can certainly lead to many broken nights.

In order to find the most suitable remedy, observe your child carefully. Is he bringing his knees up towards his abdomen? Is he bending backwards? Is he better if you carry him?

### Chamomilla

- child is **extremely irritable and complaining with the pains**
- **nothing satisfies the child or the pains**
- **better as long as he is carried**
- often accompanies teething
- may be diarrhoea, with **green stools**

### Colocynth

- pain is **alleviated by bending double or applying hard pressure** to the area
- **your child improves when he brings his knees up to his abdomen**
- better for warmth
- worse after eating or drinking

### Dioscorea

- pains are worse when the child bends forward
- **child straightens his body or may even arch backwards for relief**

### Magnesia phosphorica

- **pains are better for warm applications, warm drinks or rubbing**
- severe cramping, griping pains

### Pulsatilla

- **colic after the mother (if breastfeeding) or child eats rich foods**
- child is mild, timid, weepy; **wants affection**

Both *Pulsatilla* and *Chamomilla* may be indicated if the child cries a lot and wants to be carried. Constitutionally, the '*Chamomilla* child' is irritable and demanding with his crying. The '*Pulsatilla* baby' is more sweet-tempered and clingy, and tends to evoke more sympathy than the *Chamomilla* child.

*Potency and Repetition*

Give one dose of 12C or 30C every one to two hours, depending on the severity of the symptoms. When the pain diminishes you can increase the length of time between doses to every three to five hours. You may even find that one dose daily may be enough. If the pain continues in severity after three to four doses, and/or the relief is very short lived, another remedy may be needed and you should seek professional help.

### EXTERNAL AND COMMON-SENSE MEASURES

1 Give your child smaller, more frequent feeds.
2 If breastfeeding, the mother should avoid eating foods from the cabbage family (cabbage, Brussels sprouts, etc.). Citrus fruits or caffeinated drinks can also cause gas. Experiment with your diet and see if it affects your breast milk.
3 Nurse in a quiet, secure environment where you can maintain good physical contact with your baby. This can be calming and possibly help with digestive disorders.
4 If your baby is bottle-fed, make sure he is not sucking in too much air with his feed.
5 In older children, ginger water in chamomile tea with honey may help soothe digestion.

### CONSTIPATION

Constipation can be caused by dietary factors (such as changing from a fluid to a solid diet) or while travelling. It can also be psychological, as when a child rebels against toilet training.

Constipation comes and goes in children. If it lasts for a couple of days every now and then and there is no pain, do not worry. If persistent, or if dietary changes do not help, your child may need constitutional help.

### Alumina

◆ **difficulty passing** the **stool,** even though **soft**
◆ **constipation** after starting **on a formula**

### Bryonia

◆ **dryness** of mucous membranes
◆ **large, hard, dry stools**
◆ child can go for days with **no urge**

### Nux vomica

◆ **urging** and then, when the child passes a stool, he still **feels as if more is left**
◆ **frequent urging but passes small amounts**
◆ a **history of** taking a lot of **laxatives**
◆ **hard, painful stool, causing the child to weep as it passes**

## Opium

◆ **no sense of urgency**
◆ stools resemble **hard, round, black balls, like sheep dung**

*Potency and Repetition*

One dose of 30C three times a day for two or three days. If the constipation continuously returns, do not continue with a remedy but seek professional help, as well as trying the measures listed below.

### EXTERNAL AND COMMON-SENSE MEASURES

1  In bottle-fed babies, try changing the formula.
2  In older children, make sure they get enough fibre. Fruit, vegetables, fruit juices and exercise should help.
3  If your child shows resistance to toilet training, be gentle. Do not put too much emotional pressure on him.
4  Simmer five or six prunes slowly for a couple of hours in a few cups of water. Give your child the juice in the morning and the prunes to eat at night.
5  Avoid commercial laxatives as much as possible – they will not help the body develop its own capacity to pass stools. In some cases they can lead to more constipation in the long term.
   *If the above measures, along with the indicated remedies, do not help and the constipation does not improve after a week, seek professional help.*
6  Psyllium seeds or linusit are available in most health food shops and can be very helpful.

### WHEN TO SEEK PROFESSIONAL HELP

1  If there is vomiting, pain and no bowel movement over 24 hours, go to the hospital immediately. There could possibly be some type of obstruction.

### DIARRHOEA

Diarrhoea is a common problem with infants. As long as your child's appetite is good and there is no accompanying vomiting or weight loss, it will usually clear up by itself. You will know by the severity of symptoms whether you need professional help or not.

There are many causes of diarrhoea. Infants can often have diarrhoea when they are teething. Poor eating habits, or eating too many sweets, unripe fruits, excess ice cream can be factors, as can the frequent use of antibiotics. Bad meat or food poisoning can cause simultaneous vomiting and diarrhoea. Sudden upsets or frights can lead to this problem, and diarrhoea is also common among visitors to countries where the standard of hygiene or the quality of the water is poor.

## Aethusa

◆ during teething
◆ during summer
◆ **diarrhoea caused by an inability to digest milk**
◆ **weakness**

## Aloe

◆ **whenever the child passes wind, he passes stools**
◆ lots of wind
◆ child has a sense of **insecurity of the rectum**. He feels he has to hold on tight to stop himself from having an accident

## Arsenicum album

◆ commonly used for **'traveller's diarrhoea'**
◆ **sudden extreme weakness and exhaustion**
◆ **thirsty**, needing frequent small sips of a drink
◆ chilly
◆ vomiting and diarrhoea together
◆ after bad food
◆ **anxiety**, with a possible fear of death
◆ **burning pains**
◆ worse after midnight
◆ **combination of weakness, anxiety, chill and thirst**

### Chamomilla

- diarrhoea accompanied by painful **colic**
- during teething
- **offensive green, slimy stools, resembling spinach**
- child is **extremely irritable** and complaining, **nothing satisfies** him
- rotten egg odour to the stools

### China

- **watery, painless diarrhoea with much wind**
- child **wants to be carried**

### Colocynth

- colicky **pain which is better for hard pressure, bending double or lying on abdomen**
- worse after eating or drinking

### Cuprum

- diarrhoea where no symptoms are clear, but **cramps** are the most apparent

### Ipecacuanha

- diarrhoea accompanied by continual extreme **nausea**
- **frothy green stools**
- no thirst
- clean or pink tongue

### Nux vomica

- **after overeating**
- child **strains** and passes small amounts of stool
- **feels temporarily better after each stool**

### Podophyllum

- **worse in early morning**
- **profuse, explosive, squirting diarrhoea with lots of rumbling noises and wind**
- stool **comes out forcefully** in a shot, like water from a fire hydrant
- offensive stools
- worse after eating
- intense cramps (may cause the child to double up with pain)
- **diarrhoea**, and drooling (from the mouth) **during teething**
- during summer
- prolapse of the rectum during bouts of diarrhoea

The traditional books stress that *Podophyllum* stools are extremely offensive. We have often missed prescribing this remedy because this symptom was not present. Our experience has shown us that sounds in the abdomen and noisy, spluttering explosive stools are more important symptoms. If these are present, this is enough to indicate *Podophyllum.*

### Rheum (Rhubarb)

◆ extreme **acidity** in the stomach
◆ **stools** and whole body **smell sour**
◆ during teething
◆ child has little appetite and not much need for sleep

### Sulphur

◆ **offensive stools with no other symptoms**
◆ **anus may be red**

### Veratrum album

◆ **vomiting and diarrhoea together**
◆ very **cold sweat**, icy, pale face and tip of nose
◆ exhaustion
◆ severe cramps
◆ rapid, feeble pulse

*Potency and Repetition*

Give one dose of 12C or 30C every half hour to every two hours depending on the severity and frequency of the diarrhoea. As soon as there is a marked reduction in the frequency of the stools, give one dose after each stool. Three to four doses should be enough if the remedy is well chosen.

**EXTERNAL AND COMMON-SENSE MEASURES**

1  Avoid eating heavy, rich foods.
2  Add a cup of rice to six cups of water and simmer for one hour (add water as necessary so it does not dry out). Strain and keep the liquid. Add salt and drink it. You can give your child a cup of this drink every few hours.
3  Let your child eat yoghurt and bananas, which are easy to digest.
4  Avoid sweets, cold foods and sugared drinks.

### JAUNDICE

This occurs quite frequently in children; it normally resolves itself in a week. You should, however, always seek professional help.

Five or six doses of *Chelidonium 6C* may help this condition resolve itself without complications.

### POISONING

Should your child accidentally ingest poison, try to identify what it was, if possible. Seek immediate help at the hospital; prompt action may help avert potentially serious problems. Do not assume that because your child does not show symptoms he is out of trouble.

### VOMITING AND NAUSEA

Vomiting can be caused by a wide variety of things, quite apart from contaminated food. It can be associated with earache, worms, injury or even a respiratory problem. However, it is not uncommon for young babies to regurgitate small amounts of milk after a feed. This can sometimes be worse during teething, and is usually nothing to worry about.

If your child has severe colic and/or diarrhoea as well as nausea, please refer to these sections as well. You may find a more relevant remedy there.

If the vomiting is associated with a respiratory disorder or a childhood disease such as whooping cough, refer to these relevant sections.

## Aethusa

◆ intolerance **of milk, with vomiting of curdled masses**
◆ extreme vomiting, rapidly making the child **weak and sleepy**

## Antimonium crudum

◆ thickly **coated, milky white tongue**
◆ child **vomits after eating and drinking**
◆ loss of appetite
◆ after overeating or too many rich foods
◆ **irritability**, aversion to being touched or looked at

## Arsenicum album

- child is **extremely restless, constantly shifting around**
- **anxiety**
- weakness that comes on suddenly
- vomiting and diarrhoea together
- **bad food or water**, or ptomaine poisoning
- **thirst for frequent sips of cool drinks**, which may then be brought straight back up
- child feels chilly, desires warmth
- **burning pains, better for warmth**
- often worse after midnight (around 2 to 3 a.m.)

## Bryonia

- all complaints made **worse for any motion**; child prefers to keep completely still
- **dryness** of mouth with **thirst for large amounts of water**
- child wants to be left alone
- bitter taste in the mouth
- **worse for fatty or rich foods**

## Ipecacuanha

- **continual nausea and vomiting**, not made better by being sick
- extreme nausea
- usually **worse after eating**
- **clean or pink tongue**
- colicky, griping pains around navel
- **vomiting after coughing**

## Nux vomica

- lack of appetite
- irritability
- after overeating
- child **feels as if he would like to vomit but can't**

## Phosphorus

- **thirst for cold water**
- child often vomits once this water warms up in his stomach
- **burning pains**
- child desires company

## Pulsatilla

- child **vomits after eating fats, rich foods, ice-cream or fruit**
- no thirst
- bitter taste in the mouth
- child is often shy, and wants affection

## Silica

- infant **brings up breastmilk**
- projectile vomiting

## Veratrum album

- **vomiting and diarrhoea together**
- **cold sweat, especially on forehead**
- weakness

*Potency and Repetition*

Give one dose of 12C or 30C every one to two hours, depending on the severity of the symptoms. After their intensity has lessened somewhat, you can give the remedy every three to four hours. In most cases four to five doses should be enough. If relief is gained after the first dose, but your child then has a relapse, give him one dose each time he vomits. If there is no relief of symptoms or your child keeps relapsing even after three to four doses, this usually means that the situation calls for a constitutional remedy, or that the remedy needed is not listed in this book. Seek the help of a professional homoeopath.

**WHEN TO SEEK PROFESSIONAL HELP**

1  If your child becomes dehydrated
   In babies and toddlers, signs of dehydration are sunken eyes and fontanelles (the soft spot at the top of the head), loss of skin tone, dry nappies (little urine is being passed), dry eyes and mouth.
   In older children, weight loss of more than 10 per cent of body weight could indicate dehydration.

2  If your child vomits incessantly, especially if what he brings up is blood-stained, or if the vomiting starts after your child has sustained a head injury.
   If your child exhibits any of the following:
3  If your child seems extremely sleepy over a prolonged period of time (six to 12 hours)
4  If your child screams or cries inconsolably for longer than five hours
5  If the stools are black
6  If pain comes on rapidly
7  If constipation is prolonged and accompanied by vomiting and signs of pain or distress
8  If you have any reason to suspect your child has swallowed poison or drugs
9  If the abdominal pain is severe

### Earache

The ear is divided into three parts:

1  The external ear canal, into which children sometimes put small objects.
2  The middle ear, which consists of the eardrum and an air-filled cavity which has a tube (called the eustachian tube) connecting it to the mouth. This tube helps keep the pressure balanced between the air inside and outside the ear.
3  The inner ear chamber, involved in transmitting sound waves to the brain.

Most common problems affect the external and middle ear.

External ear problems can occur after swimming, or when children put small objects into their ears. Boils and eczema can also cause problems with this part of the ear.

Middle ear inflammation is called *otitis media*. This condition can be acute or chronic. It can flare up as a complication of tonsillitis, flu, whooping cough, measles, sinusitis or a cold. Some children have inflammation of the middle ear without these other problems. The inflammation may or may not be accompanied by a build-up of pus or catarrh. Sometimes pus and catarrh can fill the eustachian tube and produce pain, loss of hearing, bulging of and sometimes damage to the eardrum. Fluid build-up behind the ear drum can cause the ear drum to burst. This can be a thick and at times bloody discharge. It will usually heal by itself if there are no complications.

Chronic otitis media is a recurrent inflammation of the ear. It is found in an increasing number of children these days. The condition known as glue ear can develop as a result, especially where there have been repeated courses of antibiotics.

Both acute and chronic middle ear inflammation respond extremely well to homoeopathic treatment. If your child has had repeated doses of antibiotics and still has recurrent ear problems, do not hesitate to seek constitutional treatment from a professional homoeopath. Good homoeopathic treatment usually prevents the need for tubes or grommets to be inserted.

The first three remedies listed below are generally useful only in the early stages of otitis. If they seem appropriate and are given early enough, they can often stop an attack.

### Aconite

◆ at the outset for **sudden, painful** earache accompanied by **restlessness,** fear and **anxiety**
◆ after exposure to **cold, dry wind**
◆ if the ear is red and hot
◆ worse at night

### Belladonna

◆ for **sudden**, painful onset
◆ often affecting the right ear, but not necessary if other symptoms fit
◆ **bright redness** of face and/or affected ear
◆ dry, **burning skin with fever**
◆ glazed eyes, dilated pupils
◆ no thirst, and irritability

### Ferrum phosphoricum

◆ **at the beginning**; sometimes accompanied by pink cheeks and **no characteristic symptoms**

## Calcarea sulphurica

◆ if the ear drum has burst and there is a **continual thick creamy discharge of pus**

## Chamomilla

◆ **extreme sensitivity** to the pain
◆ child is very irritable and difficult to please with the pain
◆ **nothing satisfies the child, yet he continues to be demanding**
◆ child is weepy in a **rude, demanding, irritable** way
◆ **extreme pain**
◆ red cheeks, or one cheek red and the other pale
◆ pain worse for warm things

## Hepar sulphuris

◆ irritability with **extreme pain**
◆ **sensitive to cold air and cold applications**
◆ possible relief from warm applications

## Mercurius vivus

◆ often associated with swollen glands
◆ pain extends to the face and teeth
◆ sweaty, **worse at night**
◆ **offensive mouth odour**
◆ **profuse saliva** – may dribble onto pillow at night
◆ shooting pains
◆ smelly, possibly bloody discharge from the ear

## Plantago

◆ for earache **associated with toothache**

## Pulsatilla

◆ child **cries with the pains**
◆ child is **clingy, feels better if held, pampered or rocked**
◆ pains usually worse at night
◆ often prefers cool air
◆ if thirsty, prefers cool drinks
◆ thick creamy yellow, possibly greenish discharge

### *Potency and Repetition*

One dose of 30C every half hour to every two to three hours for three to four doses, depending on the intensity of the pain. There should usually be some relief after the first couple of doses.

### WHEN TO SEEK PROFESSIONAL HELP

1 If your child is drowsy, has a stiff neck, headaches and a high fever
2 If the pain continues for more than 24 hours
3 If the bony area at the base of the ear becomes painful or red (possible mastoiditis)

### EXTERNAL AND COMMON-SENSE MEASURES

1 A couple of drops of Mullein Oil (*Verbascum*) every few hours in the affected ear. Mullein oil is available at most health food stores or chemists which sell homoeopathic remedies.
2 If your child gets repeated earaches after swimming, you may have to stop him from going until you have been to a professional homoeopath for treatment. The remedies will build up his body's natural resistance.
3 Equal drops of *Plantago* mother tincture and warm water. Put a few drops into his ear every hour for several hours. This may help the remedy along. If your child also has toothache, a few drops on the affected tooth will help.

## Case Study

A 20-month-old boy started having health problems at the age of about eight months. He had a history of coughs, colds, swollen tonsils and ear infections; he had frequently been prescribed antibiotics.

Five months before coming for homoeopathic treatment, tubes (grommets) had been inserted in his ears. He had nevertheless suffered with eight ear infections since that time, along with chest complaints.

The night before our first consultation he was pulling at his ear and was complaining of pain. Once again, he was given antibiotics.

The morning of the homoeopathic consultation his right ear drum burst and was leaking a thick, gluey discharge.

He is an extremely friendly, outgoing child who can also play happily by himself for long periods of time. He is afraid of large dogs, and of falling. He does not feel the heat, but tends to be hot and hates direct sunlight.

We prescribed several doses of *Calcarea sulphurica 200*, a year later he has needed no further antibiotics. He rarely gets colds, and has had no ear problems.

What homoeopathy can do in the treatment of both acute and chronic otitis media is really wonderful.

### Exam Nerves

Some children get anxious before exams to such an extent that it almost seems to make them ill. One of the following remedies may be of help.

#### Anacardium
◆ **the child's mind goes completely blank as he sits to write, he is so lacking in confidence**

#### Argentum nitricum
◆ **hurried, anxious, irritable and nervous before exams**
◆ diarrhoea before events
◆ may crave sweets

#### Gelsemium
◆ **weakness and trembling before events or exams**
◆ may have diarrhoea

#### Picric acid
◆ **for the good student who has studied hard but cannot take any more** – he may even want to throw his books away
◆ he **fears his mind will 'let him down'** during the exam
◆ **exhausted from studying**

*Potency and Repetition*

One dose of 30C the night before the exam, one dose the morning of and another just before the exam.

## Eye Problems

Mild eye complaints can be treated at home. It is important, however, to remember how delicate the eyes are. If you are the least bit uncertain, seek professional help immediately.

### CONJUNCTIVITIS

This is also known as pink eye or sticky eye. It is an inflammation of the delicate lining that covers the eyeball. It can be caused by allergy or infection.

Allergic pink eye can be brought on by pollen, dust, chlorine in swimming pools, chemicals and pollution. The eye becomes itchy, red and weepy.

Infectious pink eye can have either a bacterial or viral cause.

In both cases the eyes are red and itchy. Viral conjunctivitis is accompanied by a clear, thin discharge; the bacterial kind produces a thick, creamy discharge.

Your child may come home complaining of a gritty, sandy feeling in his eye. He may even have swollen glands and a fever.

Repetitive or allergic conjunctivitis needs the help of a professional homoeopath.

### Apis mellifica

◆ **burning**, stinging eye pain
◆ **better for cool applications; worse for warmth**
◆ possible puffy **swelling** of the eyelids

### Argentum nitricum

◆ thick **pus-like, creamy discharge**
◆ **swollen red** lids and eyes
◆ this remedy often useful in babies
◆ **better for cool applications**
◆ sensitivity to light

### Arsenicum album

◆ **burning inflammation, better for warm applications**
◆ restlessness and anxiety
◆ acrid excoriating discharge

## Belladonna

- for sudden **intense onset**
- **very red** and bloodshot eyes
- **sensitivity to light**

## Euphrasia

- **red eyes with acrid, burning tears – the tears may redden the cheeks**
- **sensation of sand or grit in the eyes**

The common name for this remedy is Eyebright. It is used both in herbalism and homoeopathy. It can be used as an external lotion for many eye complaints as well as internally.

## Ferrum phosphoricum

- **inflammation at the outset; few other marked symptoms**
- child feels as if bits of dirt or grit are trapped under the upper eyelid

## Hepar sulphuris

- **thick, pus-like discharge;** eye pain **worse for cold**

## Pulsatilla

- **thick, bland, yellow-green discharge**
- **better for open air and cool applications**
- the child is often weepy and needing of affection

## Rhus toxicodendron

- **eyes stick together at night**
- tears rush out when the child opens his eyes first thing in the morning
- **sensitivity to light**
- painful eyes, made worse by motion
- **general restlessness**

### *Potency and Repetition*

One dose of 12C or 30C every three hours for four to six doses. Stop the remedy when the eye starts to get better; repeat it if improvement slows or ceases.

**COMMON-SENSE AND EXTERNAL MEASURE**

1 Do not let your child rub his eyes.
2 Do not share towels or flannels if the infection is contagious.
3 Use clean linen (not sponges) every time you clean the eye.
4 Moisten the eye with a cloth or eyebath to help remove stickiness. Use a solution of 5 drops of rose water and 5 drops of *Euphrasia* mother tincture in half a cup of warm sterilized water. If rose water is not available, use 1–2 drops of *Euphrasia* in an eyebath of sterilized or distilled warm water.
5 If the infection is caused by an allergy, try to discover what your child might be allergic to and remove it from his diet or environment.

**WHEN TO SEEK PROFESSIONAL HELP**

1 For any loss of vision, including blurred or double vision.
2 If the eye has been injured.
3 If the pain is severe.
4 If your child's eyes hurt in bright light.
5 If the pupils are irregular sizes.
6 If any chemicals have gone into the eye:
   *wash well with water while seeking help.*
7 If the lid or surrounding skin is extremely swollen with a yellow-green discharge.

### STYES

These are small boils or pimples that occur on the eyelids. Your child may rub his eyes or complain that it feels as if something is stuck in his eye. A small red inflamed spot appears that becomes filled with pus and eventually bursts.

## Apis mellifica

◆ **burning, stinging, swollen eyelid**
◆ **better for cool applications; worse for warmth**

## Hepar sulphuris

◆ stye slow to come to a head
◆ **very painful and sensitive to touch and to cold applications**
◆ pain may be better for warm applications

## Lycopodium

◆ **affecting the right eye, especially towards the inner corner**

## Pulsatilla

◆ **the major remedy if there are only a few symptoms**
◆ for styes affecting the upper lid
◆ pus turns yellow-green

## Staphysagria

◆ may appear after suppressed anger
◆ **styes form hard lumps**
◆ **recurrence** of styes, or repeated crops of styes

### EXTERNAL AND COMMON-SENSE MEASURES

1 Bathe the eye with quite warm water to help the stye come to a head. Do this several times a day.

### WHEN TO SEEK PROFESSIONAL HELP

1 If vision becomes distorted
2 If the stye persists for more than a couple of days despite bathing and using one of the above remedies
3 If there are systemic symptoms, such as fever and fatigue, or if the stye points inwards towards the eyeball

## Fever

Normal oral temperature is 37°C (98.6°F). Rectal temperature is 0.5°C (1°F) higher; fever taken from the armpit is 0.5°C (1°F) lower. Infants may have a slightly raised temperature in the evenings. This is normal and is not necessarily a cause for alarm. Fever is nature's way of helping your child's body fight off disease; unless it is extremely high or complicated by other factors, this is actually beneficial and not a cause for worry. Fever is not a disease but a result. Make yourself familiar with the section below on when to call for help.

There are three major types of fever:

1  A sustained fever: constantly high
2  An intermittent fever: falls back to normal, particularly in the morning, and rises in the evening
3  Relapsing fevers: feverish episodes marked with one or two days of completely normal temperature, then fever again

Along with constitutional homoeopathic treatment, here are some suggestions for parents to help a child who develops repeated fevers. The best counsel is not to expose your child to sudden changes in weather or temperature. Do not overdress him or introduce sudden changes in his diet.

The remedies listed below are beneficial for most simple, uncomplicated fevers. Fevers often precede earache, respiratory problems or childhood contagious diseases, or may accompany teething and flu (influenza). When and if other symptoms arise affecting specific parts of the body, please refer to the relevant section(s) of this book.

When looking for the correct homoeopathic remedy, it is not only the fever that is to be observed. It is what kind of fever and how your child behaves when ill that is important. The aim is to cure your child, not simply to reduce his fever. A positive change after a remedy may not take the form of the temperature dropping straightaway, but your child will seem better in himself, or perhaps his appetite may return. If your child falls asleep shortly after taking a remedy, this is a good sign. The fever should then improve.

Some of these remedies are often indicated at the beginning of contagious childhood diseases. If this is the case the remedy will not effect a cure, but will make your child more comfortable during the course of the disease. If the problem proves to be one of these diseases, refer to the relevant section of this book.

**EMERGENCY:**
## Aconite
◆ sudden, rapid onset, accompanied by high fever
◆ exposure to cold, dry weather
◆ child is **very restless, anxious, fearful**
◆ child is **dry, hot and thirsty**
◆ **rapid pulse**
◆ fear often accompanies an Aconite fever, or the fever can start after fear

## Belladonna
◆ sudden, rapid onset, accompanied by high fever
◆ **bright red, flushed face**
◆ **dilated, shiny pupils; eyes red**
◆ **skin burning hot, can feel steamy**
◆ hot head but cold feet
◆ irritability
◆ may have no sense of thirst
◆ throbbing headache

These two remedies can be difficult to distinguish at times. They both come on rapidly and are accompanied by extremely high fever; in both cases the child can become very red in the face. If *Aconite* is the required remedy, the child tends to be thirstier and is extremely fearful and anxious. If your child can speak, he may even indicate that he is afraid of dying or may ask for reassurance that he won't die. If *Belladonna* is necessary, the child tends to be more angry and irritable. His face is usually redder and his eyes may glisten.

*Potency and Repetition*
One dose of 12C can be given anywhere from every 15 to 30 minutes at first, according to the severity of the fever. If after three doses the fever has improved but tends to keep coming back quickly, give the 30C potency and repeat as needed for a few more doses. Increase the length of time between doses as your child improves.

Simple, uncomplicated fevers should respond rapidly to these remedies when they are indicated. If there is no noticeable change after an hour, another remedy may be required. Remember that a beneficial change may not take the form of an immediate absence of the fever; you may first notice that your child perks up or even starts to ask for food again, before the temperature drops.

## Ferrum phosphoricum

◆ **fever with pink cheeks** and a pale face
◆ **useful at the beginning of inflammation**
◆ fever is not as rapid or extreme as if *Belladonna* or *Aconite* were indicated; sometimes accompanied by prostration and at other times by **no marked symptoms** (however hard you look for them)

*Potency and Repetition*
One dose of 12C every half hour to every hour, depending on the severity of the experience. Three doses of this remedy is usually enough for a simple fever where there are no other marked symptoms.

**GRADUAL ONSET:**
## Bryonia

◆ **dryness** of mucous membranes
◆ **worse for all movement – child wants to keep still**
◆ slow onset, often in warm muggy weather, but possibly in cold dry weather as well
◆ child is **very thirsty**
◆ constipation, with dry stools
◆ child is irritable, wants to be left alone

## Eupatorium perfoliatum

◆ **extreme aching deep in the bones**
◆ lower back pain
◆ thirsty

## Gelsemium

◆ slow onset in warm, muggy weather
◆ child is **drowsy, lethargic, feels heavy**
◆ **drooping eyelids**
◆ **dizziness and dullness**
◆ **aching with chilliness** up and down the back
◆ child is so lethargic he **wants to lie still** and be left alone
◆ no thirst

The above two remedies are often useful for the 'flu'.

## Pulsatilla

◆ child is **weepy,** affectionate, **wants company**
◆ no thirst
◆ desires open air, **averse to heat**

## Rhus toxicodendron

◆ fever with **extreme restlessness** after exposure **to cold, damp weather** or after getting overheated and then cooling off too quickly

## Sulphur

◆ child is lazy and untidy, with a desire for open air and possibly sweets
◆ of particular use if other indicated remedies have not worked

*Potency and Repetition*

One dose of 12C or 30C every two to three hours depending on the intensity of the symptoms. Give three to four doses as needed. You may be surprised to find how often one dose will be enough.

**WHEN TO SEEK PROFESSIONAL HELP**

1 If the fever is extremely high (40.5°C/105°F).
2 If your child is less than six months old.
3 If he suffers convulsions.
4 If his neck is stiff.
5 If he suffers continuous fevers after returning from a trip abroad.
6 If within 12 to 24 hours there is no response to a homoeopathic remedy.

7 if sponging your child down with a wet cloth does not lower his temperature
8 if he has extreme difficulty breathing
9 if his consciousness is very altered, with great confusion and drowsiness

**EXTERNAL AND COMMON-SENSE MEASURES**

1 Provide open air and rest.
2 Give plenty of fluids to prevent dehydration.
3 Give him meals that are light and easy to digest.
4 Sponge his face and body down with a lukewarm wet cloth (about 18°C/65°F is suitable).
5 Cool him down with drinks of hot water with lemon and honey.
6 Help to bring the fever down with sage tea with honey, one teaspoonful to a cup, steeped for no longer than 10 minutes.

## Headache

A child's headache can be triggered by emotional upset or by stresses at home or at school. We have also noticed that eating too much 'junk food' can cause headaches as well as digestive upsets and constipation.

Children who catch a lot of colds can develop headaches across the forehead or the eyebrows, due to the pressure of catarrh.

At puberty many young girls suffer from headaches due to hormonal changes.

Headaches may also be associated with other conditions like flu or excess sun; it may be helpful to look at the relevant section(s) of this book.

Children who get frequent headaches that are not associated with acute illnesses such as flu or colds should have constitutional treatment from a professional homoeopath.

## Arsenicum album

◆ for **headaches caused by food poisoning; accompanied by restlessness and anxiety**
◆ child is chilly
◆ thirsts for frequent small sips of water

## Belladonna

◆ intense **throbbing, pulsating** headaches
◆ **onset** is often **sudden**
◆ child **can't bear light, motion, noise or being jarred**
◆ child feels worse when lying completely flat – **better when seated**
◆ face may be very flushed
◆ may be associated with a high fever
◆ pupils may be dilated
◆ pain is often right-sided
◆ head may be hot while hands and feet are cold
◆ for headaches caused by exposure to sun

## Bryonia

◆ child is **worse for the slightest motion** – even moving his eyes can increase the pain
◆ the pain **often starts on the left side** (often the left eye) and travels all over the head (possibly over the whole body)
◆ child is irritable, **wants to be left alone**
◆ may be accompanied by nausea, vomiting and constipation
◆ child may be thirsty

## Gelsemium

◆ pain **often starts on the back of the head or neck** and can extend to the forehead
◆ child feels **drowsy, dull and heavy – finding it difficult to keep his eyes open**
◆ headaches **can come from over-exposure to the sun**, accompanied by a sensation of heaviness
◆ can be associated with flus and fevers
◆ the headache **may be relieved by urinating**
◆ child is lethargic, **wants to be left alone**

## Ignatia

◆ **from grief**, loss of a loved one or a pet
◆ pain that feels like a nail in the head

## Natrum muriaticum

◆ pain feels **like tiny hammers, usually starting in the morning** and ending by late afternoon
◆ worse for sun and heat
◆ useful for **introverted children** who may be having emotional difficulties and who keep their feelings to themselves

## Nux vomica

◆ irritability with the headache
◆ **worse for overeating**
◆ worse for moving or shaking the head
◆ may be accompanied by constipation

## Pulsatilla

◆ useful for **sensitive,** weepy **children who crave affection**
◆ **may be needed at puberty**, for menstrual difficulties
◆ **worse after rich fatty foods or ice-cream**
◆ digestive problems may accompany this type of headache
◆ **better** for open air and **cold applications**

## Staphysagria

◆ useful for children who suffer from **headaches after quarrels or family upsets, especially if they suppress their emotions**
◆ for **children who are bullied at school** and have no way to express their feelings
◆ **headaches after anger**, or when anger is **suppressed**

### EXTERNAL AND COMMON-SENSE MEASURES

Cold applications at the base of the neck can relieve some headaches.

### WHEN TO SEEK PROFESSIONAL HELP

1 After an injury
   *See also* the relevant first aid section of this book (*page 23*).
2 If there is a combination of fever, neck stiffness and headache.
3 If accompanied by severe drowsiness, confusion and vomiting.
4 If there are any visual disturbances with nausea and/or vomiting.
5 For headaches that continue for more than 24 hours, or keep recurring.

## Influenza

The term 'flu' is used very loosely these days and can mean anything from a fever to a cold to true influenza. This section describes true flu. Please refer to the appropriate section for simple fevers and colds, although frequently the symptoms (and therefore the remedies) will be similar.

The incubation period for flu can be up to three days. Early symptoms are chills, fever and usually exhaustion, with aches and pains in the back and legs. These symptoms can be accompanied by sore throat, headache, cough and diarrhoea. The rise in temperature can be steep (38.9–40.6°C/102–105°F). There can also be prostration and at times delirium, which can be frightening. Your child may also be apathetic and irritable.

The duration of uncomplicated cases is usually up to seven days. However, in some cases the fatigue, sweating and weakness can last several days longer, and sometimes the exhaustion can hang on for weeks.

In the winter there are often epidemics of influenza, and they can be accompanied by ear complaints and bronchitis. If such problems occur, refer to the relevant sections of this book.

Some children have a tendency to recurrent influenza. Constitutional homoeopathic treatment is highly recommended.

### Aconite, Belladonna and Ferrum phosphoricum
◆ may be **useful at the outset.** *See* **Fever.**

### Gelsemium and Eupatorium perfoliatum
◆ **used very frequently for the flu.** *See* **Fever.**

### Arsenicum album
◆ exhaustion
◆ **restlessness** and anxiety
◆ child is **thirsty** for small sips of water
◆ **chilliness**
◆ burning pains

## Baptisia

- rapid onset with **sudden prostration**
- flu accompanied by **digestive disorders,** diarrhoea
- **aches, offensive breath**
- dull, red, drugged look
- high fever, child falls asleep while talking to you

## Bryonia

- **thirsty; dry**
- **worse for all motion**
- **wants to be left alone**
- stitching pains in chest

## Dulcamara

- after exposure to **cold, wet weather**
- **profuse mucus** discharges
- frequent urination

## Nux vomica

- child is extremely chilly, **must keep warm**
- **chilly on slightest motion**; lies under blanket and even the slightest motion causes chilliness
- chilliness after drinking

## Oscillococcinum

- **useful at the very beginning of a fever (flu), when there are few other symptoms**
- this remedy has been found to be useful in 200C potency

## Pulsatilla

- no thirst although feverish
- **prefers open air; averse to heat and stuffy rooms**
- **mild**, weepy, wants company

## Rhus toxicodendron

- great **restlessness** after exposure to **cold, damp**

## Sulphur

♦ **tendency to relapse**
♦ **flushes of heat** with desire for open air, but averse to draughts
♦ feet burn, child wants to keep them uncovered
♦ **drowsiness**

### Potency and Repetition

One dose of 12C every two to four hours depending on the severity of the symptoms. Lengthen the amount of time between doses as improvement sets in. Give the required remedy for a couple of days if necessary. Different remedies may need to be given at different stages of the illness.

#### WHEN TO SEEK PROFESSIONAL HELP

1  If there is a severe, exhausting respiratory problem (this may indicate pneumonia).
2  If diarrhoea persists.
3  If there is continuous ear pain.
4  If your child gets weaker and weaker.

#### EXTERNAL AND COMMON-SENSE MEASURES

*See* **Fever**

## Mouth Problems

#### MOUTH ULCERS

Some children seem to have a tendency to mouth ulcers. Other contributing factors can be fatigue, exams, family stress, and fever. Although the following remedies may help with an attack, constitutional treatment will often prove necessary. Consult a professional homoeopath.

Your child will probably complain of a burning, tingling feeling in his mouth. If you look inside you may see little, swollen white ulcers with red borders.

**THRUSH**

This shows up as white or creamy coloured patches in the mouth. It is particularly common in young babies. The tongue and the insides of the mouth may swell, causing considerable distress. Homoeopathy can be very helpful with this.

Depending on the symptoms, there are some remedies that can be used to treat both mouth ulcers and thrush. We have grouped them together here for your convenience.

### Antimonium crudum

◆ thick **milky white coating on the tongue**

### Arsenicum album

◆ raw red or bluish **burning ulcers, made better for warm drinks**
◆ child is restless, anxious, craves company

### Borax

◆ one of the most frequently used remedies for both conditions
◆ results are especially marked for ulcers
◆ marked fear of downward motion
◆ **pain in the mouth when sucking or eating**
◆ **hot** ulcers which **may bleed**

### Chamomilla

◆ when the symptoms of the remedy are present (*see* **Materia Medica**)
◆ child is **irritable; nothing satisfies** him
◆ **loose stool**

### Kali muriaticum

◆ **white ulcers or thrush if there are no clear symptoms to guide you to one of the other remedies**
◆ **especially indicated at the beginning of an attack**
◆ **tongue** may be 'patchy', with a **grey or white coating at the base**

### Mercurius vivus

◆ **offensive breath**, sore mouth
◆ **lots of salivation**; dribbles on the pillow

## Sulphur

◆ painful and **burning mouth ulcers, especially if other remedies have not helped**
◆ **offensive mouth odour** (when there are no other symptoms and *Mercurius vivus* has been given but has not helped)

*Potency and Repetition*
One dose of 12C or 30C every three hours for four to six doses. Once you notice the beginnings of improvement, stop the treatment or increase the length of time between doses.

**EXTERNAL AND COMMON-SENSE MEASURES**

1  Gargle with a solution of 20 drops of *Calendula* lotion to half a cup of sterilized water. You may use golden seal (*Hydrastis*) instead of *Calendula* if you prefer.
Golden seal is sometimes a very effective mouth wash for these conditions.

**WHEN TO SEEK PROFESSIONAL HELP**

1  If the ulcers or thrush keep coming back.
2  If the condition is extremely severe and painful.
3  If pus starts to be produced.

## Skin Disorders

Skin diseases cause a great deal of anxiety for both children and their parents. Homoeopaths see most problems on the skin as a result of an internal disorder. We therefore prefer to treat them with internal remedies rather than simply using external ointments to get rid of the skin eruptions, in part because we often find that, if a skin disorder is treated only with an ointment, another problem soon appears somewhere else in or on the body.

**BOILS**

Boils are inflamed, painful red bumps with a central core of pus. They can occur anywhere on the body, but often appear on the neck, face and buttocks. If your child tends to suffer from recurrent boils, he has a chronic problem that should be addressed by a professional homoeopath.

## Anthracinum

- for very **severe** boils
- **burning pains**
- **dark blood** oozes from the boil

*Potency and Repetition*

One dose of 30C every three to four hours for three to four doses.

## Arsenicum album

- **burning pains, better for warm applications**

*Potency and Repetition*

One dose of 30C every three hours for three to four doses.

## Belladonna

- at the outset of an attack, before pus has formed
- boils are **red and hot, accompanied by throbbing pain**

*Belladonna* is only useful for boils if it is given within the first few hours of inflammation. Once pus has even started to form, it will rarely be of any value.

*Potency and Repetition*

One dose of 12C or 30C every one to two hours, depending on the intensity of the symptoms, for three or four doses. If *Belladonna* does not resolve the inflammation, try one of the following remedies.

## Hepar sulphuris

- for boils that are **slow to form a head**
- extremely **painful**
- **sensitive to touch and cold applications**

*Potency and Repetition*
One dose of 6C every one to two hours for four to five doses. If this remedy is correct there will be fairly quick relief from the pain.

## Silica
♦ **slow to heal after the pus has been discharged**

*Potency and Repetition*
One dose of 12C or 30C every three to four hours for two to three days.

## Sulphur
♦ for **repeated boils**
♦ slow to heal
♦ useful for *Sulphur* **constitutional types**

*Potency and Repetition*
One dose of 30C every three to four hours for three doses.

## Tarentula cubensis
♦ for large boils accompanied by **extreme burning and stinging pain**
♦ when the boils are **purple**

*Potency and Repetition*
One dose of 30C every two to three hours, depending on the intensity of the symptoms, for three to four doses.

### EXTERNAL AND COMMON-SENSE MEASURES
1 Soak the boil(s) with a hot compress to help bring it to a head and discharge.
2 Some people have found that honey mixed with a small amount of flour and applied as a poultice can be helpful.

### WHEN TO SEEK PROFESSIONAL HELP
1 If the boils recur over and over again.
2 If they are accompanied by fever and/or swollen glands.
3 If there is no improvement within two to three days.

### COLD SORES

These are caused by a viral infection and take the form of tiny blister-like eruptions in and around the mouth and/or lips.

The attacks can be mild and may sometimes be accompanied by a slight fever. If your child has recurrent cold sores, constitutional treatment from a professional homoeopath is the best strategy.

You may try one of the following two remedies to help for acute attacks.

## Natrum muriaticum

◆ for herpes that come on after **exposure to hot sun**
◆ sometimes known as 'fever blisters'

## Rhus toxicodendron

◆ after **exposure to cold, damp weather**

*Potency and Repetition*

One dose of 30C every three hours for four to six doses.

### CRADLE CAP

Many infants develop cradle cap – a crop of thick, crusty, scaly, yellow eruptions on the head and around the ears. It is nothing to be overly concerned about and usually clears up of its own accord. If you would like to treat your baby's cradle cap, however, the following remedies may be useful. Sometimes a constitutional remedy such as *Calcarea carbonica* may be of help; please consult a professional homoeopath.

## Mezereum

◆ for crusty **eruptions** that **ooze from under the crust** especially when slight pressure is applied

## Sulphur

◆ **offensive smell on the head, with no other symptoms**
◆ inoffensive smell to the cradle cap, but strong-smelling stools/urine

*Potency and Repetition*

One dose of 12C or 30C every 12 hours for three doses.

**EXTERNAL AND COMMON-SENSE MEASURES**

1 Coat the scalp with coconut oil or a non-medicated cream overnight to moisten and help soften the scales. You can gently remove some of the scales, but do not pull them off.
2 Do not be tempted to use a hard brush on your baby's scalp to get rid of the cradle cap.

**ECZEMA**

This is a skin disorder characterized by itching and redness. In severe cases the symptoms can be extreme and may be accompanied by cracks, bleeding, and weeping of anything from a thin watery discharge to a thick honey-coloured fluid.

In some children the skin thickens where it itches most, particularly in folds of skin as at the elbows, knees, and the groin.

Orthodox medicine has come round to the view (long held by homoeopaths) that eczema can be caused by hereditary factors, sensitivity to certain foods, allergies, emotional states or a combination of all four. We usually do not recommend home treatment, but suggest that you consult a professional homoeopath. The use of a skin cream or lotion rarely deals with the underlying cause and, although it may provide relief, this is usually only temporary.

**EXTERNAL AND COMMON-SENSE MEASURES**

1 Avoid dairy products.
2 Limit your child's intake of any foods or substances he seems sensitive to.
3 Applying coconut oil or a bland non-medicated cream on areas of thickened skin may help soften the skin.
4 Avoid wool, man-made fabrics, strong soaps and anything that may irritate the skin.

### Case Study

Linda brought her six-month-old son, Oliver, for homoeopathic treatment for his eczema. His skin was very dry and he had cradle cap as well. On a general level he was a happy baby who slept well and was just beginning to eat solids. He was suffering from slight constipation, which could possibly have been attributed to the change from just milk to solid foods. Linda's pregnancy and birth had been uneventful, and Oliver had had no immunizations to date.

We first gave Oliver *Sulphur 30*. Over the next three months, however, his eczema did not improve. We decided to prescribe *Graphites 200*, but there was still no change. The doctor at the local health centre did not want to prescribe steroid creams for such a young child, and was sympathetic to homoeopathic alternatives. The most obvious symptom at our third interview was a delay in the start of teething. The homoeopathic remedy *Calcarea carbonica 200* was prescribed; within one week Oliver's eczema was clearing from his face, and his first teeth had come through. To date his eczema has improved significantly, to the delight of his family and doctor.

Homoeopaths often see dramatic responses like this when the correct constitutional remedy is given. It is interesting to note that we did not spot the correct remedy straightaway. This demonstrates that should you ever make a similar misdiagnosis, giving your child the incorrect remedy cannot do him any harm.

### Case Study

An 11-month-old boy was brought by his parents for skin problems, diagnosed as eczema. The symptoms we noted were as follows:

- His parents had been using cortisone cream on his skin regularly, with only temporary benefit.

- The red eruptions were very bad around his nipples, and were discharging a clear to reddish fluid. The dry patches on other parts of his body were very itchy.

- He had had four colds since his birth and had been treated with antibiotics three times.

- His nose was stuffed up and his chest would be very congested at times.

- His hands and feet were cold; he was also feverish.

- He would get 'yeast' rashes quite frequently.

- He was generally an easy child, not crying a lot.

- He was very hyperactive, alert, getting into everything. Liked to explore. He was all over the place in the clinic while his case was being taken.

- He had started walking at nine months old.

- Sleep was a problem: after a broken night, though tired he would still try to get up out of his cot.

- Would move his hands and feet while asleep. Slept in the knee-to-chest position.

Taking all these symptoms into consideration, we gave him *Medorrhinum*. There was an immediate but consistent improvement of his skin complaints over the next six months, as well as a noticeable reduction in the number and frequency of his colds and chestiness.

With chronic skin complaints the whole child has to be taken into account.

### HIVES (NETTLE RASH)

This skin disorder is characterized by raised areas of hot red skin, often in blotches, accompanied by severe itching and swelling. Hives can be caused by allergies, shellfish, spices, sweets, drugs or insect bites. Recurrent hives usually need constitutional treatment.

#### Apis mellifica

- **itchy** red blotches **worse for** heat, **warm applications, and** possibly **at night**
- worse after exercise, perspiration or **when overheated**
- after insect bites or bee stings
- **better for cool applications**
- **swollen skin, can feel as if it will burst**

### Arsenicum album
◆ **hot,** red eruptions **better for warm applications**

### Rhus toxicodendron
◆ **itching that can be soothed by the application of very hot water**

### Urtica urens (Stinging nettle)
◆ this remedy comes from the stinging nettle
◆ nettle rash appearance
◆ raised, **red, burning blotches**
◆ **worse at night, for warmth, when overheated**
◆ after eating shellfish

*Potency and Repetition*

One dose of 12C or 30C every three hours for three doses. As with all homoeopathic treatment, stop once your child shows signs of improvement.

**EXTERNAL AND COMMON-SENSE MEASURES**

1  Apply cool applications.

**WHEN TO SEEK PROFESSIONAL HELP**

1  If the respiratory tract gets affected and breathing becomes difficult.
2  If there is a history of severe reactions to similar causes.

**IMPETIGO**

This is an infectious skin disorder that is common in children. It is extremely contagious. Playgroups and schools will exclude a child with impetigo until it has completely cleared up.

The eruptions can occur anywhere on the body, but usually form on the face and legs. They are usually seen around the lips, and can resemble cold sores.

Impetigo starts off as elevated spots containing yellow pus. The spots then break open and form crusts. Scratching can spread the infection to other parts of the body.

Homoeopathy can usually treat impetigo quite successfully. Antibiotics are rarely necessary.

If the following remedies do not work there are others that probably will and which might relate more to the constitutional symptoms of your child. Consult a professional homoeopath.

### Antimonium crudum

◆ typical **picture of impetigo – thick, yellow-crusted eruptions on the cheeks and chin which weep and ooze**
◆ may be a thick white coating on the tongue
◆ child is miserable and difficult to get along with

### Arsenicum album

◆ **burning, itching eruptions better for warmth or warm applications**
◆ restlessness

### Graphites

◆ **eruptions are thick, oozing a honey-like discharge, accompanied by scabs**
◆ child may be chubby (this is a constitutional symptom)

### Mezereum

◆ **glue-like discharge oozing from thick crusts, especially when the crusts are pressed**
◆ redness around the eruptions

### Rhus toxicodendron

◆ extremely **itchy, especially at night**
◆ child is **restless,** cannot keep still
◆ eruptions may feel **better for hot applications**

### Viola tricolor

◆ thick scabs with a thick yellow pus
◆ itching with burning, worse at night

*Potency and Repetition*

One dose of the indicated remedy in 6C or 12C every three to four hours for up to six doses. If the remedy is correct your child should feel better generally within 24 hours, even if the skin does not yet look better.

**EXTERNAL AND COMMON-SENSE MEASURES**

1 Avoid contact with other children.
2 Wash the crusts with warm sterilized water and *Calendula* lotion (approximately 10 drops of *Calendula* to half a cup of water). Do this several times a day.
3 If the eruptions are infected, wash with an *Echinacea* mother tincture solution (10 drops in an egg-cup sized container full of cooled boiled water). Do this approximately every four hours.

**WHEN TO SEEK PROFESSIONAL HELP**

1 If the above remedies do not help and your child is in great distress,
2 If there are signs of severe infection.

**MILK CRUSTS (BABY ACNE)**

Small white pustules on the cheeks and forehead. They start on the face and spread to the rest of the body. The spots can go yellow, burst and form crusts. This is a self-limiting condition which usually clears up in about three or four months. Occasionally orthodox medicine recommends antibiotics, but we have found that homoeopathic remedies are usually sufficient. If one of the following remedies does not provide relief, a constitutional remedy may be necessary. Seek a professional homoeopath for help.

Aconite

◆ at the outset; **bright red inflammation accompanied by anxiety and restlessness**

Rhus toxicodendron

◆ very **itchy**, accompanied by **restlessness**

Sulphur

◆ offensive odour to all bodily discharges (urine/stools/breath/sweat)
◆ **itching worse when the child is warm in bed at night**

## Viola tricolor

- scabs with a **sticky yellow pus**
- **itching worse at night**
- symptoms that are helped by *Sulphur* and *Viola tricolor* are worse at night. If the symptoms are strictly local and there is no offensive smell from any part of the body, try *Viola* first.

### *Potency and Repetition*
One dose of 12C every four hours for four to six doses.

#### EXTERNAL AND COMMON-SENSE MEASURES
1   Wash the eruptions several times a day with a lotion made up of 10 drops of *Calendula* mother tincture to half a cup of sterilized water.

#### WHEN TO SEEK PROFESSIONAL HELP
1   If symptoms do not improve within a few days.

#### NAPPY (DIAPER) RASH
Sometimes, however hard parents try to prevent it, nappy rash takes hold.

Sensitivity to cow's milk and soya sometimes aggravates the skin. Breast is usually best, but if that is not possible you may have to try changing your baby's formula. In some cases very severe nappy rash needs constitutional treatment. The rash may be caused by acidic urine or stool; remedies can alter their acidity. External treatment on its own will provide only temporary relief.

## Sulphur

- for a **red rash** that is **between the buttocks**, on the genitals and, often, extends up the back

### *Potency and Repetition*
One dose of 30C every three to four hours for three doses.

**EXTERNAL AND COMMON-SENSE MEASURES**

1 Apply *Calendula* lotion (10 drops of *Calendula* mother tincture to half a cup of sterilized water) a couple of times a day.
2 Expose the affected area to the air as much as possible.
3 Avoid plastic pants if possible.
4 Wash the area frequently and change wet or soiled nappies as soon as possible.
5 Make sure that the detergent you use is very mild.

**WHEN TO SEEK PROFESSIONAL HELP**

1 If the area develops a white, cheesy-like coating (thrush).
2 If the rash begins to bleed.
3 If it is very painful and persistent.

**PSORIASIS**

This skin complaint is characterized by scales that often start on the head (resembling dandruff) and on places like the elbows and knees. This scaling or flaking often leads to a thickening of the skin. This is a chronic disorder and must be treated by a professional homoeopath.

**WARTS**

Many children have warts these days and go through upsetting rituals of having them removed by a variety of different means, only to have them come back. Warts can come and go quite unexpectedly, or can crop up for a period of time and then never be seen again.

Homoeopaths treat warts as they do other skin complaints, with the use of internal remedies; we have had great success treating them homoeopathically. The remedies listed below have been known to help, though a constitutional remedy may be required if you are to eradicate the warts completely.

Antimonium crudum
♦ for warts or **hard growths on bottom of feet**

## Causticum

◆ for **fleshy** warts on the **face or around** or under **the fingernails**

## Dulcamara

◆ for large, **flat, hard and smooth** warts on the **back of the hands** or on the **face**

## Thuja

◆ for **soft, spongy, fleshy** warts, usually appearing on the genitals (though they can occur anywhere on the body)
◆ may be painful and may bleed

*Potency and Repetition*

One dose of 30C every 12 hours for three doses. Allow two weeks to a month before you consider a different remedy.

**EXTERNAL AND COMMON-SENSE MEASURES**

1 Use an external application of a few drops of *Thuja* mother tincture if you wish.

## Teething

Teething (dentition) is usually a straightforward matter. Teeth start to appear at the age of around five to eight months; by a year old most children have approximately six to 10 teeth. At 18 months there are usually 12 teeth; at two years approximately 16 to 20. By two and a half, all 20 baby teeth are usually in. Adult teeth start to come through when children are about five to seven years old.

Problems with teething include pain while the teeth are erupting, or some kind of delay or slowness in their development. Symptoms associated with teething can be as simple as loose stools and dribbling. Other indications are hot and cold flushes, chest complaints, high fevers with diarrhoea, and/or emotional states such as tearfulness and whining, fretful, restless behaviour.

The following remedies can be of help to alleviate these problems. If your child is suffering from a specific condition such as diarrhoea or a chest complaint, you may find a more suitable remedy under the relevant section of this book.

## Aconite

- **extreme pain with great anxiety, restlessness and, often, inflamed gums**
- the child may rub his gums with his fist to try to alleviate the pain
- worse for cold air or cold drinks

*Potency and Repetition*

One dose of 30C every one to three hours, depending on the intensity of the symptoms, for three to five doses. This should help 'take the edge off' the pain and ease the restlessness.

## Calcarea carbonica

- useful where there is **delayed development of** not only the **teeth** but of the bones in general – such as **slowness of the fontanelle** (the soft spot at the top of the head) to close
- *Calcarea carbonica* **is a constitutional remedy**, useful for children with a tendency to **plumpness** (they are also often fair-haired), and general slowness
- **sweaty head**
- **loose stools**, if present, are often **sour**

A calcium deficiency is often the root of the problems this remedy can cure. This is usually caused by the body's inability to assimilate calcium efficiently, rather than a lack of calcium in the diet.

*Also see Calcarea phosphorica* (below). If you think either of these two remedies is indicated, we advise you to discuss this with a professional homoeopath.

## Calcarea phosphorica

- **delayed development of teeth and** also of bony structures such as the **fontanelle** (the soft spot on the head)
- **sweaty head**
- *Calcarea phoshorica* **is a constitutional remedy**, useful for children who are thin (and often dark-haired, though not always)

*Potency and Repetition*

One to three doses of 30C every three to 12 hours. As mentioned, this is a constitutional remedy; you should discuss your child's symptoms with a professional homoeopath.

## Chamomilla

This remedy can be useful for a variety of conditions that can accompany teething, such as diarrhoea, chest complaints, pain, etc. The most important symptoms which *Chamomilla* can help, however, are usually emotional ones.

This remedy has won over many sceptics because of its quick action. It is often used routinely for painful teething. However, it works much better when the characteristic symptoms listed below are present.

- child is **whiny, irritable, stubborn and just plain miserable**
- he does not want to be bothered or even looked at
- he may even strike out with anger
- **anger with the pains**, which seem unbearable
- child is **capricious, nothing satisfies him**; he may ask for something and then immediately want something else
- he is **quiet as long as he is being carried**
- **one cheek hot and red** (usually the side the tooth is coming through on), **the other cheek is pale**
- **loose stools**
- child may have difficulty breathing; a short, hacking cough
- **worse at night**

### Kreosote

- **teeth start to decay quickly** after they appear
- child is **restless, agitated**, capricious, nothing satisfies him
- **very inflamed**, spongy or bleeding **gums**
- **severe pain**

A dose of 12C or 30C every three to six hours for a few doses should be sufficient. *Chamomilla* may also be useful for a chronic situation. If the above symptoms persist, seek help from a professional homoeopath.

### Mercurius vivus

- **excessive salivation** accompanied by offensive bad breath
- worse at night

### Podophyllum

- salivation and **noisy, explosive diarrhoea**

*Potency and Repetition*

For *Mercurius vivus, Podophyllum* and *Chamomilla*:

One dose of 12C or 30C every two to five hours, depending on the intensity of the symptoms, for three to five doses. A remedy like *Chamomilla* may have to be repeated daily for one to three doses during the period that the tooth is coming in, as necessary.

## Silica

◆ **slow development** of teeth
◆ **sweaty neck and head**
◆ child is **timid but stubborn**

*Silica* **is a constitutional remedy**, for children who are thin (and who often have **fine hair**)

*Potency and Repetition*

One to three doses of 30C every three to 12 hours. As mentioned, this is a constitutional remedy; if you think *Silica* is indicated you may wish to discuss your child's symptoms and general physical and emotional state with a professional homoeopath.

### EXTERNAL AND COMMON-SENSE MEASURES

1 Give your child something to 'gnaw' on.
2 Give him something cold and solid (like an ice-cube wrapped in a clean cloth) to chew on.

### WHEN TO SEEK PROFESSIONAL HELP

1 If the problem persists and/or relief is short-lived.
2 If symptoms include a chest complaint that keeps getting worse.

## Throat Complaints and Tonsillitis

Children frequently develop sore throats or even tonsillitis during the winter. These problems often right themselves, without the need for any treatment. Most of the time your child's own immune system will deal with the inflammation within a week.

The tonsils, two small glands at the back of the throat, exist to protect the respiratory tract from more serious complaints. When one or both of them get inflamed, this is called tonsillitis. Swollen tonsils are often associated with swollen adenoids and can cause associated hearing difficulties.

There is no orthodox treatment for the type of tonsillitis or sore throat caused by a virus. If a sore throat caused by bacteria develops into tonsillitis, with the typical swollen glands, fever and malaise, antibiotics are often the recommended treatment.

Homoeopathy is excellent for viral and bacterial tonsillitis and in many cases can prevent the need for surgery. In our years of experience we have seen that antibiotics are not necessary to the extent that most people believe. Children with throat and tonsil problems usually respond very quickly and successfully to homoeopathic treatment.

If your child has had many courses of antibiotics, homoeopathic treatment may not immediately stop the throat infections. If you persevere you will be pleasantly surprised to find a reduction in the severity and frequency of attacks. Homoeopathy helps build up your child's own natural resistance to disease.

The following remedies have been found effective for many acute throat complaints. If the problem is recurrent or if these remedies do not provide suitable relief, consult a qualified homoeopath.

The first three remedies are often indicated at the beginning of treatment. In sore throats and tonsillitis affecting small children, *Belladonna* is often the first remedy to consider. Do not give it routinely, however, without first verifying the symptoms.

### Aconite

◆ **often indicated at the beginning**
◆ **after exposure to cold, dry winds**
◆ **complaints come on suddenly and violently**
◆ child is very **anxious** and **restless**, often fearful
◆ **high fever**
◆ **thirst** for cool drinks

### Belladonna

◆ right-sided problems
◆ **very often one of the first remedies indicated for small children**
◆ **complaints come on suddenly and with great intensity**
◆ useful at the onset of a sore throat or tonsil infection
◆ **high fever; the child's head is hot, his face and throat are red, though often his extremities will be cold**
◆ sensitivity to light
◆ child desires lemonade but may be thirstless

### Ferrum phosphoricum

◆ **at the beginning, in cases where there is inflammation but very few other symptoms**
◆ pale face with pink cheeks

*Potency and Repetition*

Give one dose of 12C or 30C every half hour to every two hours, depending on the severity of the symptoms, for three to six doses. The above remedies will usually provide quick relief. Once your child is improving, increase the amount of time between doses. Often one or two doses will be enough.

Remember that if your child falls asleep after taking a remedy, this is a good sign. Let him sleep.

### Apis mellifica

◆ very **swollen tonsils** with **stinging pains**
◆ if no tonsillitis, the **throat is pink** with stinging pains and may feel as if swollen
◆ no sense of thirst, but **pain is alleviated with cool drinks and made worse by warm drinks**

### Baryta muriaticum

◆ **very hard, swollen glands** – tonsils and back of neck
◆ **hearing may be impaired** as the swelling blocks off the eustachian tubes

## Hepar sulphuris

◆ child feels **very chilly**
◆ **throat pain better for warm drinks**
◆ pain may extend to the ear on swallowing
◆ feels **as if a splinter** or fish bone is in the throat
◆ often useful when **pus** has formed with the first two symptoms

## Lachesis

◆ pain is **left-sided, or moves from the left to the right side**
◆ **worse for warm drinks** – sometimes better for cold drinks
◆ neck and tonsils very **sensitive to touch**

## Lycopodium

◆ pain is **right-sided, or moves from the right to the left side**
◆ pain usually builds up slowly

## Mercurius vivus

◆ **child is sensitive to both heat and cold** – he will lie in bed, get chilly, cover himself – then feel overheated and take his blankets off – and keep alternating in this way
◆ **perspiration** provides no relief
◆ **excessive salivation**, may dribble on pillow
◆ **offensive breath**, pus on the tonsils
◆ complaints are **worse at night**

## Mercurius iodatus flavus

◆ similar **symptoms to *Mercurius vivus***, i.e. salivation, though predominantly **right-sided**

## Mercurius iodatus ruber

◆ as above, but **left-sided**

If soreness affects only the left or right side of the throat, and this is the only clear symptom, think of the above two remedies before any others, unless there are any other symptoms which clearly point to other remedies.

## Phytolacca

- ◆ pain usually **right-sided, shooting into the ears on swallowing**
- ◆ **aching** limbs along with fever
- ◆ pain **worse for warm drinks**

*Potency and Repetition*

Give one dose of 12C or 30C every one to four hours, depending on the severity of the symptoms. If 12C gives relief but the child suffers a relapse soon afterwards, give 30C before you try another remedy. Lengthen the amount of time between doses as improvement takes place.

**EXTERNAL AND COMMON-SENSE MEASURES**

1  If your child is prone to sore throats in the winter, always make sure he wears a scarf.
2  Gargling several times a day with a mixture of 10 drops of *Calendula* mother tincture in half a glass of warm salted water can help.
3  Give your child foods that are easy to digest – you may even want to liquefy some fruit for him to drink.
4  Large amounts of Vitamin C (one gram a day or more), especially when symptoms first start, can be helpful.
5  A drink of warm honey and lemon can be very soothing.
6  Consider stopping your child from swimming for one winter while he receives homoeopathic treatment.

**WHEN TO SEEK PROFESSIONAL HELP**

1  If the pain is severe and accompanied by swelling and difficulty swallowing.
2  If the tonsils are so swollen breathing becomes obstructed.
3  If the pain persists for more than five days with no signs of improvement.
4  If respiratory problems develop along with the throat problem.
5  If the problems recur.
6  Occasionally sore throats can persist and glandular fever (mononucleosis) is diagnosed. Along with prolonged bed rest, homoeopathy can be effective in these cases.

7 the major concern from a streptococcal throat infection is the risk of developing a kidney disorder or rheumatic fever. If there is a family history of these problems, you must seek professional help whenever your child comes down suddenly with a throat infection.

## Travel Sickness

Many children get sick when travelling in cars, trains, boats and planes. It can be quite distressing. The cause can be more than just the motion. It can be the fumes, lack of oxygen, or a combination of these. Homoeopathy has several remedies that can be helpful, according to the symptoms.

Constitutional treatment may help to prevent a recurrence.

### Borax

◆ **nausea caused specifically by downward motion**

### Cocculus

◆ severe **nausea, vomiting, vertigo** and sometimes headaches **from the motion of the boat or car**
◆ **lots of salivation**
◆ worse for the sight or smell of food
◆ child **must lie down**

### Nux vomica

◆ **irritable and sick from overeating** at the beginning of the trip

### Petroleum

◆ **one of the major remedies for motion sickness where there are no clear symptoms or other remedies have not helped**
◆ headaches (often at the back of the head)
◆ child feels chilly but likes the open air
◆ **salivation**

## Tabacum

- ◆ child has a pale or green, sickly appearance
- ◆ extreme nausea and vertigo
- ◆ child **lies still, with his eyes closed**
- ◆ is chilly and in a **cold sweat**
- ◆ **needs the open air** – will go on deck or open windows
- ◆ may feel better for uncovering his stomach or abdomen
- ◆ likes to lie in the dark

## Theridion

- ◆ **nausea and vomiting worse for motion and when the child closes his eyes, especially for excitable children**

Note that children who need *Theridion* keep their eyes open, while those requiring *Tabacum* get relief by closing their eyes.

### Potency and Repetition

Give two to three doses of 12C or 30C every three hours the day before the trip if it is to be a long one. On the day of the trip, administer the remedy every two to three hours, or as needed, for three or four doses.

If it is to be a relatively short trip, give one dose a couple of hours before the trip, one when the trip starts, and another a couple of hours later if necessary.

**WHEN TO SEEK PROFESSIONAL HELP**

1  If none of the above helps.

## Umbilical Hernia

This is a protrusion of a loop of the intestine through a weakness or scar area in the navel region.

A small umbilical hernia tends to be self-limiting, but if it does not heal try homoeopathy before surgery.

### Calcarea carbonica

♦ as mentioned, *Calcarea carbonica* is a constitutional remedy for chubby children whose tissues are lax and flabby. They may also be prone to having a sweaty head

*Potency and Repetition*
One dose of 30C every 12 hours for three doses, then wait. If there is some improvement after a couple of weeks but then this improvement stops, give one more dose of 30C. As long as improvement continues, there is no need to repeat the dose.

If this remedy is not indicated or does not help, consult a qualified homoeopath.

## Worms

Some children seem to be prone to worms. However hard parents try to maintain scrupulous hygiene, the worms keep returning.

There are four main types of worms:

1 **Threadworms**: also known as pin or seat worms. They are like small white pieces of thread that can be seen crawling on the anus at night (when they come out to lay eggs). These are the most common types of worms in children.
2 **Roundworms**
3 **Hookworms**
4 **Tapeworms**

Worms live in different parts of the digestive tract, depending on the type of worm. An itchy anus, itchy nose, bloating, loss of appetite and nausea may indicate the presence of worms.

Worms, especially threadworms, can be very tenacious and hard to eradicate at times. *We recommend that if your child has frequent infestations of worms he gets constitutional homoeopathic treatment.* This will help alter the flora of the digestive tract to create a less favourable environment for the worms to live in. Remedies such as *Calcarea, Sulphur* and *Silica* may sometimes help, but should only be given under the advice of a professional homoeopath. In extreme cases where your child is in great discomfort or distress, orthodox treatment may be needed. This should then be followed up with homoeopathic treatment.

### Cina

- child is cross, **angry, irritable, nothing satisfies** him
- he constantly picks or rubs his nose
- **itchy nose and anus**
- dark rings around the eyes
- large appetite

### Granatum

- pain **around the navel**, accompanied by an itchy anus
- **hunger** and salivation

### Natrum phosphoricum

- extreme **acidity, accompanied by a yellow tongue**
- child craves sweets and starches

### Spigelia

- pain **around the navel**
- **intense crawling sensation around the anus**

### Teucrium

- when **nothing else seems to help**
- child is **restless at night**
- picks and **scratches his tingling nose**
- sensation of crawling around the anus
- **offensive breath**, loss of sense of smell

*Potency and Repetition*

One dose of 6C three times a day for one week.

### EXTERNAL AND COMMON-SENSE MEASURES

1 Avoid sugar, pastries and potatoes. Sweets provide an environment that worms seem to thrive on.

2 Give your child dry roast pumpkin seeds: about 30 to chew three times a day. Not to be taken at the same time as food.

3 Some people have found eating large amounts of garlic (raw) helps to eradicate worms.

4 Maintain good hygiene, particularly as your child may scratch the worms crawling out of the anus at night. If he then puts his fingers in his mouth, the whole cycle starts all over again. Sometimes an ointment such as Vaseline around the anus will help, along with scrupulous cleanliness.

### WHEN TO SEEK PROFESSIONAL HELP

1 If the worms seem to recur often.

2 If none of the above measures works.

# chapter six

# homoeopathic treatment of childhood diseases

The childhood diseases discussed in this chapter usually respond quite well to homoeopathic treatment. Homoeopathic treatment does not make these illnesses disappear overnight, but can prevent complications, shorten the course of the disease, and alleviate a lot of your child's distress.

These diseases often go through different stages; different remedies may have to be given at each stage. Do make sure you call your health care practitioner if your child suffers any complications.

For each illness we list the possible remedies for each set of symptoms (both the physical symptoms and ones that describe your child's emotional state). The most significant symptoms are printed in **bold** type.

## Chicken Pox

The incubation time is 14 to 21 days. Chicken pox is contagious from a few days before the onset of symptoms up until all the water-filled (vesicular) eruptions have crusted over. It may start with a mild fever, headaches, malaise and sore throat.

The rash starts as spots, which turn to vesicles that come out in crops and can linger for a few days to two weeks. These water-filled blisters then become crusty and dry up. Eruptions are rarely on the face and extremities, and usually predominate on the upper trunk.

## Aconite, Belladonna or Ferrum phosphoricum

◆ may be indicated for the fever stage at the beginning even before the spots have erupted. Please see the **Measles** section (*page 123*) for the symptoms that would indicate these three remedies

## Antimonium crudum

◆ child is irritable, **impossible to satisfy**
◆ wants to be left completely alone
◆ thickly coated **white tongue**
◆ **accompanying cough or bronchitis**

## Antimonium tartaricum

◆ drowsy, **sluggish, miserable**
◆ **accompanying cough or bronchitis**
◆ rash is slow to show itself
◆ pus-filled eruptions
◆ accompanying nausea

## Pulsatilla

◆ **weepy, needs affection and company**
◆ dislikes the warmth, likes fresh air
◆ possible lack of thirst and fever

## Rhus toxicodendron

◆ **intense itching and restlessness**
◆ **tosses and turns because of the itching**
◆ **a good remedy to consider first if itching is the only symptom**

It is important to remember that, if a cough is present, you should take this into account when selecting the right remedy. Always check the tongue to tell whether your child needs *Antimonium crudum* or *Antimonium tartaricum*.

*Potency and Repetition*
For all these remedies, one dose of 12C every three to four hours, for a couple of days.

## Sulphur

◆ often indicated **near the end if the chicken pox drags on**
◆ **itching worse when the child is warm in bed or in a warm bath**
◆ irresistible need to scratch

*Potency and Repetition*
One dose of *Sulphur 30C* every three hours, for three doses.

### COMPLICATIONS

Complications of chicken pox are rare, though should they occur homoeopathic treatment is usually quite effective. The most common are a mild bronchitis, eye inflammation, or arthritis. If none of the above remedies helps and you are worried, seek professional advice.

### EXTERNAL AND COMMON-SENSE MEASURES

1  A bland diet that is easy to digest.
2  Use no ointments to suppress the eruptions, as it is important to allow the eruptions to come out.
3  Lukewarm wet compresses may help reduce the itching.
4  Olive oil applied externally may also help the itching.

## German Measles (Rubella)

This disease has a four- to 21-day period of incubation (that is, the time between when the disease is contracted and symptoms begin to appear). Common symptoms are mild fever, malaise, and occasional joint aches. One to five days later a pinkish rash spreading from the face to the trunk appears. This rash usually lasts from one to three days. There can be swollen glands at the back of the neck under the hair line. Earache and headaches may be present but are unusual. This disease is so mild that it can be present yet hardly be noticed.

**TREATMENT**

German measles rarely needs any specific treatment, but if your child is distressed because of the fever a few doses of *Ferrum phosphoricum 12C* may be given.

The only symptoms that may need to be treated are rare complications such as earaches (*see page 75*).

The main danger with rubella is if a mother-to-be contracts it during her pregnancy. Avoid coming into contact with any child with rubella if you are pregnant, particularly during the first three months.

## Measles

This is a common childhood disease which responds well to homoeopathic treatment. The period between 'catching it' and the appearance of symptoms is seven to 14 days.

It has several stages. The infectious stage lasts from two to four days before the eruptions until two to five days after their appearance. At first measles resembles an ordinary cold, with fever, a runny nose, a cough and eyes which are sensitive to light. The eruptions appear three to five days after the cold-like symptoms start; often there is no possibility of diagnosis until the rash appears. Sometimes, but not always, there are little white spots inside the mouth (Koplik's spots) during the cold phase, which confirm that it is in fact measles.

The eruptions on the body are usually pink. They start around the ears and face and spread from there to the rest of the body. The fever usually goes up when the rash starts and then diminishes over time. The rash usually lasts for four to seven days after the eruptions appear.

### Aconite

- ◆ **sudden onset**
- ◆ **high fever, red eyes, restlessness, anxiety, fear**
- ◆ dry, barking cough

### Belladonna

- ◆ **sudden onset**
- ◆ **high fever with bright red face, red eyes**
- ◆ miserable, irritable mood

## Ferrum phosphoricum

◆ **fever at the beginning** with pink cheeks and **only a few other symptoms, if any**

The above three remedies are usually useful at the onset of the disease.

*Potency and Repetition*
These remedies can be given in the 12C or 30C potency every one to five hours for the first couple of days, depending on the severity of the symptoms. As your child's distress eases, lengthen the amount of time between doses.

### Apis Mellifica

◆ **red, puffy and hot** face/body/specific affected part
◆ **hot air aggravates the symptoms; the child prefers cooler surroundings**
◆ rash recedes early, leading to distress which can be accompanied by swelling (around the affected area or all over) or a high fever
◆ no thirst; possibly only scant urine

### Bryonia

◆ slowness of onset
◆ **moving makes the child feel worse**
◆ **thirsty, very dry throat**
◆ wants to be left alone
◆ heat makes the child uncomfortable
◆ eruptions slow to come out
◆ cough with the above symptoms, especially if the rash is slow to emerge

### Euphrasia

◆ redness centred **around the eyes**
◆ burning tears; eyes extremely sensitive to light
◆ bland discharge from nose

### Gelsemium

◆ **slowness of onset**
◆ **dull, drowsy, heavy-limbed sensations**
◆ no thirst

## Kali Bichromicum

- thick, **stringy**, almost rope-like **yellow greenish discharge** from the nose, ear, or brought up from the chest
- **mucus difficult to cough up or blow out**
- swollen neck glands

## Pulsatilla

- **weepy, clingy, wants company**
- **wants windows open, needs air**
- no thirst
- thick yellow mucus discharge from nose, possibly accompanied by a cough
- **ears may be affected**

### Potency and Repetition

The above remedies can be given in the 12C potency every three to five hours for up to six doses. Either stop the remedy or lengthen the time between doses as your child improves.

## Sulphur

- child feels worse in the heat of her bed
- red, pinkish complexion
- weakness and fatigue
- **rash slow to come out or disease slow to finish**

### Potency and Repetition

One dose of *Sulphur 30C* every three hours for three doses.

### COMPLICATIONS

The eruptions can stop coming out and cause deeper distress. There can be severe eye discomfort. There is also a possibility that coughs, catarrh or ear problems may continue after the disease seems to have run its course. Very rarely, measles can be fatal. This is more common in non-Western countries where children face continual problems of poor diet and generally poor health. In case of any complication, if none of the above remedies helps or if you are concerned about your child's progress, do seek professional advice and help.

### EXTERNAL AND COMMON-SENSE MEASURES

1 Keep the room dark, especially if your child's eyes are particularly sensitive to light.
2 If the fever is high, gently washing your child down with a wet cloth can help alleviate her distress. Do this only if the fever is extremely high. The fever is an essential part of the measles as it helps the eruptions come out.

## Mumps

Mumps is a contagious disease causing painful enlargement of the salivary (parotid) glands. Mumps is rarely seen in children under two and is usually not a serious problem. The only difficulty can be when it strikes boys after they have reached puberty, when it can affect the testicles. Infants up to one year are usually immune.

The incubation period is 14 to 24 days. Symptoms include chills, lack of appetite, headache and fever, which may last up to 24 hours before the glands under the ears swell. This swelling makes the child look like a chipmunk storing food. The temperature may rise when the glands swell. Swelling generally reaches its maximum severity on the second day and is usually finished within a week. The swelling usually starts on one side, subsiding just as the other side starts to swell up.

### Aconite, Belladonna and Ferrum phosphoricum

◆ may be useful at the onset of mumps
◆ refer to the **Measles** section for a list of the leading symptoms that would indicate one of these remedies.

### Pilocarpus jaborandi

◆ **dry mouth accompanied by salivation**

This remedy is one of the best for mumps, even when there are no characteristic symptoms. Usually hardly any other remedy is necessary.

*Potency and Repetition*
One dose of *Pilocarpus jaborandi 6C* every three hours for three to six doses.

## Lachesis

◆ **left gland swollen** and extremely **sensitive to** the slightest **touch**

## Mercurius vivus

◆ extreme **sweat and salivation**
◆ extremely offensive mouth odour

## Pulsatilla

◆ **swollen testicles** (just one or both)
◆ child feels worse for heat, better for cool
◆ likes company, feels weepy

## Rhus toxicodendron

◆ left-sidedness of swelling
◆ **cold, damp aggravates the symptoms**
◆ restlessness

*Potency and Repetition*
One dose of 12C every three hours for three to six doses.

### COMPLICATIONS

Inflammation of the testicles can occur in adult males or boys who have reached puberty if they have not had mumps previously. This can affect fertility, so seek professional help.

### EXTERNAL AND COMMON-SENSE MEASURES

1  A diet that is easy to chew and digest will help reduce the pain of eating.

## Whooping Cough

This childhood disease has a seven to 14 (sometimes 21) day incubation period. It is probably the most frightening of all childhood diseases, because the coughing fits can be so distressing to a child (and her parents!).

The disease goes through three distinct stages:

### STAGE ONE
The catarrhal stage is characterized by sneezing, listlessness, loss of appetite and a hacking cough. This cough is frequently worse during the night. Whooping cough can be very contagious during this phase.

### STAGE TWO
After 10 to 14 days the cough usually becomes paroxysmal. About five to 15 quick coughs in succession followed by a deep, hurried in-breath. This in-breath is accompanied by a noise which is the characteristic 'whoop'. This coughing fit subsides and then the whole pattern starts all over again. During this quiet interval, which is usually short but can be lengthy, your child may show no real distress. There may be large amounts of very thick chest mucus. The eyes can go red and in some cases there may even be a nosebleed as a result of the coughing. Vomiting and gagging also often accompany the cough. These symptoms can cause a lot of stress for everyone involved. Weight loss, dehydration and convulsions can also occur.

### STAGE THREE
The convalescent stage starts around the third to fourth week as the coughing fits lessen in frequency. In some cases the cough may return over the following months, after exposure to pollution or due to other upper respiratory tract problems.

Whooping cough can be serious in children under two. It can also be quite hard to have to stand by and watch your child go through the distressing coughing fits. During a fit it may seem as if your child will never breathe again – she may even turn a bit purple due to a lack of oxygen. Although whooping cough can go on and on, homoeopathy has a good track record when it comes to treating it. Different remedies may have to be given for the different stages. Although you may wish to try to treat this yourself, we would strongly advise you to consult a professional homoeopath for practical as well as emotional support.

Properly chosen homoeopathic remedies can ease your child's distress significantly, shorten the duration of the disease, and prevent or reduce the effect of any complications.

Vaccination does not guarantee immunity from whooping cough. A type of 'masked whooping cough' can develop in vaccinated children, making diagnosis even more difficult. Such children may develop a cough which goes on and on, with the occasional feeble whoop.

The following remedies are classified into the relevant stages, for ease of reference. If the symptoms would seem to indicate a particular remedy they can be given to your child no matter what the stage.

### STAGE ONE

### Aconite

◆ **sudden onset of high fever, accompanied by anxiety and extreme restlessness**
◆ barking cough, especially around midnight, accompanied by anxiety

### Arnica montana

◆ violent, tickling cough
◆ **child often cries before the cough starts, in anticipation of it**
◆ blood vessels in the eyes redden from the exertion of coughing
◆ may also be useful in other stages if indications are present

### Belladonna

◆ **sudden onset of high fever, usually accompanied by irritability**
◆ dry, barking cough, worse at night, accompanied by a **bright red face**
◆ head feels as if it will burst
◆ dryness of larynx, causing spasmodic cough
◆ child may grasp at her throat

**STAGE TWO**

## Coccus cacti

- **large amounts of very thick white mucus** which the child finds very difficult to expel
- mouthfuls of thick, foamy white mucus
- paroxysmal coughs, particularly in the morning, producing stringy white mucus
- **child prefers to be kept cool**
- cool water may halt the paroxysms if given as they begin
- **retching, accompanied by coughing**

## Corallium rubrum

- violent, **dry, spasmodic coughs, in quick succession**
- blueness of the face, accompanied by the cough
- exhaustion from the cough

## Cuprum metallicum

- extreme exhaustion from the exertion of the rapid coughing fits
- **child clenches her thumbs**; whole body goes rigid **during coughing fits**
- **child coughs and coughs until she has no breath left, then lies totally rigid, her face blue, as if lifeless**
- convulsions accompanied by above type of symptoms

## Drosera

- **Hahnemann's main remedy** for whooping cough
- coughs follow one another in quick succession
- cough **starts as soon as the child lies down**
- hoarse, barking, metallic, **deep sounding** cough
- nosebleeds accompany the cough
- abdominal pain on coughing – child may put her hand under her rib cage, where the pain is centred
- talking, singing and laughing aggravate the cough
- child **vomits** thick mucus **on coughing**

## Ipecacuanha

- bleeding from the nose or mouth during the coughing fit
- nausea and vomiting accompany the cough
- wheezing and spasms accompanied by a blueness in the face
- **a combination of bleeding, nausea and wheezing** are strong indications that this remedy is what is required
- convulsions accompanied by stiffness, loss of breath and a blue face
- pink tongue, not coated as you might expect; a lot of saliva

## Veratrum album

◆ cough accompanied by **great weakness** and **cold sweat on forehead**

**STAGE THREE**

## Antimonium tartaricum

◆ **coarse rattling of mucus in chest, very difficult to bring up**
◆ eating and anger aggravate the cough

## Pulsatilla

◆ thick yellow mucus, especially if your child is **clingy, weepy**
◆ **child prefers cool, open air; dislikes heat**

### *Potency and Repetition*

One dose of 30C potency for all of the above remedies, every three to four hours for four to eight doses (depending on the severity of the symptoms).

## Sulphur

◆ **if convalescence is slow**
◆ child is tired, lazy, averse to being overheated

### *Potency and Repetition*

One dose of *Sulphur 30C* every three hours for three to four doses.

**COMPLICATIONS**

You should definitely seek professional help for whooping cough.

1  Serious complications are rare in children over two years old.
2  Otitis media (middle ear inflammation) is very common. Some of the above remedies may help – *see also* **Earache** (*page 75*).
3  Should convulsions or acute bronchitis arise please seek professional help.
4  A cough can keep recurring for as long as a year – if so, do seek professional advice.

### A Note about Vaccination and Homoeopathic Prevention

The debate between those who favour vaccination and those who oppose it, or at least have reservations about it, has been going on for many years. The orthodox view is that vaccination has helped to conquer the life-threatening epidemic diseases such as smallpox and tuberculosis. Vaccinations are said to help control diseases such as tetanus, measles and whooping cough, as well as epidemics of influenza which can put people (particularly the elderly) at risk of more serious complications.

This short discussion is related primarily to the vaccinations given for measles, mumps, German measles (rubella), and whooping cough. We have had experience with these, not with the other diseases for which vaccinations are commonly recommended.

It is not the purpose of this book to deeply enter into the 'for or against' debate about immunization. At the end of the day, parents must make the decisions that they feel most comfortable with. However, with regards to the major prevalent childhood contagious diseases, homoeopathy has proven time and again to be very effective.

Most of you reading this book will remember being ill with the measles, missing school and then going back without any major problems. There are some schools of thought that believe that when children acquire these diseases they can actually strengthen and develop their immune system. There are certainly some children who respond poorly to vaccinations. Complications these days tend to be more common in children who already have a weakened constitution, a poor diet, or who live in unhygienic conditions.

For over a hundred years homoeopaths have been carefully observing their patients on an individual basis, noting what affects them and how. It has been observed many times that acute or chronic complaints appear to date from the time when a person was first immunized against a particular disease. In our experience we have seen recurrent fevers, ear problems, coughs and colds that have developed after the DPT, MMR and other vaccinations. These symptoms were not there before the child had the vaccinations. Little actual research has been done either to support or refute these claims. The evidence for this comes instead from the case files of individual homoeopaths.

While there are homoeopathic remedies that are used as preventatives, no official research data has verified homoeopathic beliefs. Many homoeopaths have observed that the prophylaxis listed below seems to help during epidemics. These remedies have not always arrested the illnesses in question, but have greatly alleviated the intensity of symptoms and reduced the severity of complications when compared with those experienced by other children not given homoeopathic preventatives.

Some homoeopaths do not like to give remedies prophylactically (as a preventative measure). They prefer to wait until the disease is present and prescribe on the basis of specific symptoms as they appear. This is very much an individual decision, to be made by you and the practitioner together.

If you are concerned about immunization, there are books and organizations (such as The Informed Parent) that can help you make a decision. (Please see the Useful Addresses and Further Reading chapters.)

### Homoeopathic Prophylaxis

We suggest that, if you want to give your child homoeopathic preventatives, they be given as follows (at the time of the relevant epidemic). For more advice and if you want more information on any illness not included here, please consult your homoeopath.

| | |
|---|---|
| Chicken pox | Varicella 30 |
| German measles | Rubella 30 |
| Measles | Morbillinum 30 |
| Mumps | Parotidinum 30 |
| Whooping cough | Pertussin 30 |

Give one dose of the relevant remedy (for whichever illness you are trying to prevent) 12 hours apart for three doses the first week (i.e. three doses over 24 hours). Follow this up with one dose the following week and continue to give one dose weekly during any epidemic of the relevant illness.

Thankfully, epidemics of these illnesses never seem to coincide. In any case, never give your child remedies for two of these illnesses at the same time.

# chapter seven

# treatments for newborn babies

These remedies have been found useful for newborn infants. They are not the only appropriate ones, but seem to be the most commonly indicated. See also the relevant sections elsewhere in this book. Some of these conditions will require professional help. These remedies may be useful before, while or after your baby receives it.

### Blueness

Blue babies who are cold, especially if they are also experiencing respiratory or heart problems – *Laurocerasus 30*: one dose every two to three hours, for three or four doses.

*Carbo vegetabilis 30* in the same way if *Laurocerasus* does not help.

### Colic

*see* **Digestive Problems** (*page 64*)

### Constipation

If the mother has had a lot of anaesthetics during delivery, this can lead to constipation in the newborn. One dose of *Opium 30C* every three hours, for three or four doses.

*See* **Constipation** (*page 67*) for other remedies.

## Diarrhoea

One dose of *Aconite 30C* every two to three hours, for three or four doses, especially if the baby also has a fever.

*Rheum 30C* in the same way if your child smells sour and his stools are sour.

*Sulphur 30C* every three hours for three doses if your child has offensive diarrhoea with no other symptoms.

Do not worry too much if your child has loose stools. It is common for breastfed babies to have loose stools several times a day. They are usually only a problem in newborns if accompanied by excessive weight loss, loss of appetite and/or vomiting.

## Fright

After a fright – three doses of *Aconite 30* if accompanied by restlessness.

*Opium 30* in the same way if *Aconite* does not help.

Fear may be due to invasive treatment (even just injections) during labour, or may be the baby's reaction to being left alone in an incubator.

## Injuries to the Neck and Spine During Delivery

One dose of *Hypericum 30* three times a day, for two days.

## Milk, Sudden Aversion to

*Silica 30* – one dose every 12 hours, for three doses.

*Lac defloratum 30* in the same way if *Silica* does not help.

If there are specific problems like vomiting after a feed, *see* **Digestive Disorders**.

## Sleepy Babies

This term here applies to babies who show no signs of alertness whatsoever. They may be so drowsy they find it difficult even to feed.

*Opium 30* – one dose every three or four hours, for three or four doses.

For sleepiness that is an after-effect of shock: *Aconite 30* – one dose every six hours, for three doses.

## Snuffles

Snuffles are caused by a thickening of the membranes in the nose, producing a mucus discharge that makes it difficult for the infant to breathe or feed. If the following remedies are of no help, seek professional homoeopathic help for constitutional treatment.

*Sambucus nigra* is useful where the **nose is dry and blocked,** where there is **difficulty breathing while feeding or nursing,** or when **the baby wakes suddenly, almost suffocating.** One dose of 30C three times a day, for two or three days.

*Nux vomica* – **nose dry and stuffed up at night, nose runs more freely during the day.** If *Sambucus nigra* has not helped, try *Nux vomica. Nux vomica* does not usually apply if the sense of suffocation while feeding is present – in such cases, *Sambucus nigra* is the remedy of choice.

One dose of *Nux vomica 30C* three times a day, for two or three days.

Stop repeating either *Nux vomica* or *Sambucus nigra* once your infant starts to get better.

*Pulsatilla* – **snuffles accompanied by a thick, yellow, creamy catarrh.** One dose of 30C every four hours, for three or four doses. This remedy is particularly useful in children who are **generally mild and are better for being cuddled.**

## Sore Eyes

If the inflammation has been caused by **too much light or oxygen in the incubator**: one dose of *Aconite 30C* every six hours, for two or three days. Discontinue the dosage when relief is obvious.

*Belladonna* – **red eyes, swollen lids and watery eyes**: one dose of 30C every three hours, for three to five doses. *Belladonna* is also useful if *Aconite* does not help.

*Argentum nitricum* – **eyes are red with a creamy discharge**: one dose of 30C every four hours, for three to five doses.

Give *Sulphur 30* where there is a **profuse creamy discharge** and *Argentum nitricum* does not help: one dose of 30C every four hours, for three to five doses.

## Urine Retention

One dose of *Aconite 30C* every three to four hours, for three or four doses.

Urine retention is often accompanied by screaming and crying before urination.

*Pulsatilla 30C* (one dose every three to four hours, for three or four doses) if *Aconite* does not help.

# section three

homoeopathy
and your child's
emotions

# chapter eight

# your child's emotional development

The purpose of this chapter is twofold:

A  to discuss failure to thrive in children of any age, and how homoeopathy can help
B  to introduce parents to some behavioural difficulties that can be treated effectively with homoeopathy.

**For these problems we do not recommend that you treat your children yourself,** but rather that you seek the advice of an experienced homoeopathic practitioner. When you consult a homoeopath about the types of problems discussed in this chapter, you will be prescribed what we call 'constitutional treatment'. This means that your child's current mental and emotional states are taken into account as well as her general state of health.

## Failure to Thrive

Some babies and children just do not develop properly. All sorts of advice may have been given on nutrition and general management. In spite of all this, and after full medical investigations, no cause or underlying disease may be found. This situation would also encompass cases where there are neurological problems, but no clear diagnosis. Affected children can range from being marginally slower than average when it comes to reaching certain developmental milestones (starting to talk, walk, etc.) to having serious learning disabilities.

Failure to thrive can be due to genetic factors, birth trauma, environmental changes or social or cultural problems. It is such a huge topic that homoeopathic treatment is really only recommended in certain situations. For example, slowness in walking, talking or teething, in homoeopathic terms, can often be simply a problem related to the body's ability to take in calcium. In our experience, when we have prescribed homoeopathic constitutional treatment for this type of case the clinical evidence shows that the homoeopathic remedies appear to strengthen the nervous system, build immunity, and improve the child's rate of development to bring it back within the 'norm'.

## Matthew's Case

Matthew was 10 years old and had a history of constant sore throats, swollen glands and tummy aches, as well as fever, sometimes accompanied by delirium or vomiting and diarrhoea. He had no stamina and was very thin. He slept well and loved his food, especially spaghetti, burgers and spicy dishes, but he never put on any weight. His bowels and urine were normal but he had very sweaty, smelly feet. He had difficulty keeping up with school work as he was continually ill, but he worked very hard to stay level with the rest of his class.

### HISTORY

Matthew had been a small baby. At four months he had his first stomach upset with vomiting and diarrhoea; since that time there had been several episodes of this problem. At 18 months he started to develop ear infections; he had had approximately six courses of antibiotics a year up until the age of 10 (about 60 courses in all!).

He was always worse during the winter and never put on weight. When his mother brought him to the homoeopath, Matthew said, 'I am constantly getting sick in one way or another and I feel dreadful.' In spite of this he was cheery and outgoing, though his mum said he could be quite self-sufficient and didn't seem to have any fears.

Matthew was prescribed *Silica.*

Three months later, his mother reported that he had generally been well. 'He went skiing for one week with no health problems. He now rarely gets sore throats and tummy upsets. He used to be off school for one or two weeks at a time every month, but since starting homoeopathic treatment he has only missed the occasional day. The sore throats he gets are not progressing to tonsillitis as they normally would. His appetite is good and he is putting on weight.'

Over the next year Matthew continued to improve and did not require any more antibiotics. His mother said, 'It's a miracle. In the past we didn't go anywhere without antibiotics, we had them all the time just in case, because he was ill every few weeks. He somehow could never thrive and get over his sickness. Now he is better – even his sweaty feet have cleared up!'

### SILICA

Children who need *Silica* usually lack stamina physically, mentally and emotionally. The homoeopathic literature describes the child needing *Silica* as 'lacking grit'. They can be charming and well behaved, but may have their own views which they keep to themselves. They frequently suffer from repeated colds, tonsillitis and swollen glands, especially around the ears and neck.

### Imogen's Case

This five-year-old child had suffered recurrent colds, fevers and chest infections since her third birthday. She also had continuous ear infections, swollen glands and chronic catarrh. She was generally well in the summer months, but within days of returning to nursery school in the autumn she would catch colds again. She seemed to have no resistance to anything that was going around. In her short life she had also had two severe bouts of bronchitis and had been on repeated courses of antibiotics. Sometimes when suffering from these colds she would also vomit.

She was a cheerful and sociable child when she was well, but even then her appetite was poor and she was afraid of the dark and suffered with nightmares. We prescribed *Tuberculinum.*

Three months later the report from her mother was that Imogen had been much better and her appetite had improved. There were no fevers or colds, only a small infection that did not need treatment.

Seven months after starting homoeopathy, Imogen was generally well. She was sleeping better and her nightmares had gone. She still caught colds and suffered from catarrh, but they only lasted a short time and did not require antibiotics. Her mother said she was now hyperactive and craved salty foods, ice-cream and spicy food. We recommended *Phosphorus*.

Imogen has now had seven years of homoeopathic treatment and her mother reports that her health has been excellent even through the winters. She is calmer and sleeps well. Even when all the other children are sick at school Imogen only catches the odd sniffle, and has not used antibiotics in all the time we have treated her with homoeopathy.

Imogen's case is typical of the sort of improvements that we expect with homoeopathy when long-term treatment is undertaken. To achieve these results you must go to a qualified practitioner who can prescribe the correct homoeopathic remedies, at specific intervals, to promote long-term health.

### TUBERCULINUM

Children needing this remedy suffer frequent relapses of any condition that affects them, have swollen glands, and catch colds easily. This treatment may only be prescribed by a homoeopathic practitioner.

### PHOSPHORUS

Children who need *Phosphorus* are affectionate and lively. They may suffer from fears and nightmares, as well as a tendency to frequent colds and chest infections.

## Behavioural Problems

In our society we pay a lot of attention to physical and mental development. There are many children's books on the developmental milestones. What is often missed is that children also go through more subtle, emotional developmental stages.

Our aim here is to introduce you to some of these stages, and to recommend homoeopathic treatment where appropriate. We make no attempt to give an in-depth view, but would refer you to the Bibliography (*page 214*) if you find this particular line of approach interesting.

### Anxiety, Fears and Crying

Most of us assume that when a baby is born it experiences the world somewhat similarly to the way we do as adults. However, the mind of a baby simply receives impressions and sensations, either pleasurable or distressing; he has no concept of time or space. The baby is learning in the first few months the limits of his body. As the infant approaches one year of age, his senses develop, moving beyond this state of 'primal innocence'.

It is quite possible that until the age of approximately four to six months, the child may not even realize that it is separate from his mother. The beginning of recognizing that one is separate from one's caretaker may be the start of the development of the so-called ego or personality. Understanding your infant's world will help you to deal with difficulties that may confuse you as your infant starts to grow. More and more evidence shows that some unhappy early experiences can in some cases have serious long-term consequences. A better understanding of the world of the child could help us to avoid such consequences.

Obviously babies are vulnerable and need protection. Instinctively at times of distress they will prefer to have their mother cuddle and comfort them, but up to the first few weeks, in some cases, they are happy to be comforted and held by anyone. However, by around six months the baby clearly prefers those he is familiar with – his parents or primary carers as well as his brothers, sisters or grandparents.

Separation distress is a normal part of child development: at around six to eight months a baby may react positively, or at worst neutrally, to a stranger – but by 12 months some babies will more than likely burst into tears if a stranger tries to pick them up or come too close.

For there to be 'separation anxiety', the child must realize that he is separate from his mother. This 'loss' of the person who protects him can seem devastating to a child. Many parents, seeing their once happy and contented baby suddenly reduced to an anxious, tearful bundle, can feel helplessly confused.

When a child reaches this stage, unfamiliar situations can seem very scary unless his mother or someone familiar is there. It is at this time that lengthy separations (over days) can be excruciatingly difficult for the child, and if at all possible should be avoided. The child has no experience of time, remember, so his mother's absence will seem to him final and for ever. If you have to leave your baby for several hours a day, as most working mothers do, the best solution is to make suitable, consistent arrangements for leaving him with someone he has come to know and trust; a routine of this kind will help him to feel secure.

When you are introducing a new childminder or babysitter to your child, give him a chance to bond to the new person while you are still there with them. Do not hurry your child up towards independence. It is better that your child discovers independence for himself.

There will always be children who cry and worry more than others. Here we are talking about the crying and anxiety that are not related to something obviously wrong, such as hunger, thirst, wet nappies, loneliness or pain. Constitutional homoeopathic treatment can help in situations where anxieties and tearfulness escalate into excessive states of clinginess or crying. Homoeopaths may use such remedies as *Pulsatilla, Phosphorus, Calcarea carbonica* or *Staphysagria*. These help children to feel calmer, enabling them to work through the miseries and anger that events in daily life bring.

Older children often suffer from specific fears. These can include fear of the dark, of animals, ghosts, crowds, strangers, thunderstorms, new situations and loud noises. Nightmares, sleep-walking and teeth-grinding are other ways that anxiety manifests in children. Homoeopathy helps settle these emotional upsets, especially if other, daytime difficulties are also recognized and addressed.

### Jane's Case

Jane, aged four, came for homoeopathic treatment for asthma. She was very afraid of the dark, of ghosts, and of loud noises. Her mother went out to work and was aware that being away during the day contributed to Jane's fears. Arranging a good childminder after school was essential to help with the separation anxieties. Jane also received the remedy *Phosphorus* as constitutional treatment. Her asthma improved, and her parents found that Jane became more confident and that her night-time fears diminished.

### Grief and Loss

When a mother has to go away for a long period of time, having already established herself as the primary carer, a child may experience feelings of abandonment. This may reveal itself in the child's protestations, despair and detachment. Children do not know about time until they reach about six years of age; saying 'I'll be back in two days' means nothing to them. Around the ages of two, three or four, if the mother disappears for a few weeks, at a core level it may feel to the child like she has gone for ever.

In 1953 a psychotherapist called Robertson made a special study of the despair that sets in when children up to the age of about 24 months are separated from their mothers. He found that some children became frantic with grief, experiencing the absence of the mother probably as we experience the death of a loved one. The young child has no way of knowing how to deal with this loss. We do not know if children have any notion of death, but the sense of loss can trigger deep panic and depression, and the child may be thrown into insecurity.

If we can begin to acknowledge the feelings children might have at times of separation and do the best we can to provide secure alternative care, this can help to make the situation less traumatic for them. It is a fundamental error to think that the child is 'just being naughty' if he plays up in misery or anger during and after times of separation. This behaviour may be his only way of expressing and/or managing his sense of loss.

The psychotherapist John Bowlby also carried out an in-depth study of children receiving long-term care in hospital. He found that their yearning for their mothers lingered on and on. Initially children would cry intensely for the first few days, particularly around bed-time. In some cases they would even try and search for their absent mother. As the days went on, the children's behaviour changed, though their despair remained apparent. At a later stage some children appeared to lose interest in their mothers and became emotionally detached from them. Other children when returned to their families were found to be excessively clingy, apparently fearing that if they lost sight of their mothers they would be separated again, and as a consequence of this displayed anxious behaviour.

It was mainly through Bowlby's observations of children that we finally came to recognize how important it is that mothers stay with their children during any hospital treatment.

Protest, despair, grief, mourning and detachment are defence mechanisms, and these responses are just phases of a single process. If you begin to understand this process, your child's 'clinginess' or 'difficult behaviour' can start to make sense and to be seen in its greater context. This recognition, along with the correct use of homoeopathy, can help to restore the trust and love of life that a child naturally possesses.

When a primary carer disappears either through illness, death or divorce, it can be deeply disturbing and confusing to a child. The various emotions are normal responses to these situations. Where homoeopathy can help is when you notice that there have been long-term changes in the emotional behaviour of your child, such as disruptive moods or withdrawal. We have found that remedies such as *Ignatia*, *Natrum muriaticum* and *Aurum metallicum* can be useful in these circumstances.

Do not forget that if you are really having problems with your child after a death or a separation, you should make every effort to get some family therapy or short-term bereavement counselling to help you deal with your child's distress as well as your own.

## Anger, Hyperactivity and the 'Naughty' Child

There is a whole range of behaviour which is perfectly natural and normal, so what is deemed 'naughtiness' must be seen in the context of a particular family's dynamics.

Families that provide love, security and boundaries as well as honesty and consistency of care can understand the child's misbehaviour in the greater context with his need to mature.

When a child is growing up he pushes away at the boundaries on all fronts; what you do as an adult to contain or control his behaviour is crucial, as you can ameliorate or exacerbate the situation. There is no doubt that children need boundaries; the form they take will depend on your culture and your own up-bringing.

Some children at a very early age are aware of naughtiness, but may not yet have developed a part of themselves that can control this behaviour. As children mature they become aware of the notion of choice in connection with behaviour; it is at this point that you may find your battles becoming less intense, as the naughty behaviour settles down and your child is more open to reasoning (until he hits the teenage years!).

When dealing with what you think is naughtiness in your child, try not to take it personally, do not blame and punish, but rather limit and try to contain and love. We know that there are often some very trying developmental stages, but it is important to remember that these exasperating phases will pass. Remember, your child is not some vicious demon to be curbed, but just someone who has not yet learned the social and behavioural limits we all must learn to adopt. It is quite natural to feel very angry with your child. You may even occasionally have frightening fantasies about hurting him. If you can put yourself into 'neutral' you will find your child's behaviour far easier to deal with than if you react with hatred or fury. By all means, grant yourself the anger at the irritating behaviour of your child, and if it does overwhelm you make sure afterwards that you can show your child that you still love him.

## Tom's Case

Tom's case is typical of the type of behaviour where homoeopathy can help.

At two-and-a-half, Tom was going through his tantrum phase. He was dictatorial and restless, and would sometimes hit both his parents. He would shriek for attention and then wail. At other times he would be very affectionate and, as his mother described him, 'cuddly'. Both his parents were bewildered as to how to deal with his behaviour; whatever they offered him he did not seem to want. He was given the remedy *Chamomilla,* and four weeks later his mother reported that he seemed much happier in himself, that the tantrum phase seemed to have passed and that, in addition, his general physical health (he had previously suffered from recurrent catarrh and a cough) was excellent.

### CHAMOMILLA

Children needing *Chamomilla* tend to be very irritable and are satisfied with nothing whatsoever except being carried in their parents' arms. They can have tantrums and may strike out at anyone who seems to annoy them.

At the age of approximately two, a child's struggle for autonomy begins. He wants more independence and the chance to explore his surroundings on his own. Quite often the average child will only obey half of his parent's commands at this stage; this can be extremely frustrating for the parent. It is important to know that this is simply a phase that will be passed through.

It is often around this age that a sibling is born, so apart from the difficulties your toddler has in discovering his sense of self and others, he has to deal with the feelings of jealousy. These feelings need acknowledging – punishing them simply does not help. Try to reinforce your child's good behaviour, praising him lavishly when he does something well, and minimizing your reactions to any behaviour that arises out of jealousy.

## Simon's Case

Simon was a much-adored child whose baby brother Sam was born when Simon was just two-and-a-half. Simon developed nightmares and a strong fear of the dark. He was prescribed a remedy called *Stramonium*, and his mother was warned that there would be a very angry outburst of temper, perhaps lasting a few weeks, which would be in reaction to what Simon could only view as the intrusion of his new brother. His jealous feelings had been expressed through his nightmares, so we now fully expected to see a day-time expression of this behaviour as the remedies began to help Simon adapt to the changes occurring in his life. We told his mother not to leave the two children alone together.

Simon's feelings did indeed become very aggressive towards his baby brother, whom he would attempt to hit and squash. After three weeks, however, the whole situation calmed down. Simon was still feeling jealous, which is what you would expect, but his desire to hurt his sibling had abated.

It is very interesting to note that as soon as Simon started openly expressing his anger, his nightmares and fear of the dark completely disappeared. The explanation of this is that even young children learn early which behaviour is acceptable (that is, will meet with mum and dad's approval) and which is not. Simon did not openly express his anger about the injustice of having a new rival for his parents' affection. Instead this anger turned into something that was feared, and then the nightmares started. Once he felt safe to express his anger during the day-time, the nightmares no longer had a psychological purpose, and so disappeared.

Jealousy is normal. If it gets out of hand, however, that is the time to seek out the help of a qualified homoeopath.

### STRAMONIUM

This is a remedy for children who are tremendously fearful in the night, especially when they are alone. They can wake in terror from nightmares, clinging to or calling anyone who is nearby. During the day they are often bad-tempered, or can alternate between being quite mild and agreeable and very aggressive.

There are some children, however, whose behaviour persistently transgresses their parents' set boundaries for no obvious reason which anyone can understand. The child who is consistently aggressive when there appears to be no underlying psychological reason for this antisocial behaviour might be helped with homoeopathy.

Hyperactive children can have sweet natures or be obstinate and bossy. Some can be so restless that they will not sit down for meals, run around continually and can even behave quite nastily, instigating quarrels just to let off steam. It is quite likely that, if the reasons for a child to act this way cannot be found within his family situation, there may be some undiagnosed chemical imbalance contributing to this manic activity. This is just the kind of problem homoeopathy is good at addressing. We have treated many cases where children have benefited from constitutional homoeopathic treatment. We find in these cases that, although the child's fundamental character does not change, he can be helped to be much more calm and reasonable.

## Some Strategies for Dealing with Your Child's Moods

1 We all have moods, and so do children. Try not to feel responsible if your child is in a bad mood. You do not have to do anything about it. His mood will change. If you like, you can try to find ways of involving your child in something else to take his mind off his bad mood.

2 Be firm, objective and try hard not to get caught up in your child's moods. Try to be a stable and secure presence, and if there is something your child seems to be trying to tell you, try to be open to it and to respond to it constructively.

3 Boundaries must be firm. For example, if your child is angry because he cannot get something he wants, such as a sweet, do not let him wear you down. If you cannot bear the noise, leave the room (so long as it is safe to leave him where he is). Take a deep breath and stay away for a few minutes, checking periodically to make sure that your child is safe. Return only when you have calmed down. If you are in public, trying to

reason with your child will not work. The best you can do is either hold the child or, again, wait as quietly and calmly as possible. Know that you are good enough and that you are doing the best you can. There is always a part of you that cannot bear your child's behaviour. In those infuriating moments when you are also feeling angry, try to keep bearing it. Good enough is good enough!

4 Find out if there is a pattern to the mood swings. Hunger and fatigue can easily set a child off. See if you are pushing yourself beyond your own limits. If you are feeling upset due to overwork, your child will pick up on this and react to it.

5 Discuss your child's difficulties with a homoeopath to find out whether the problems are suitable for homoeopathic treatment.

# section four

homoeopathic
remedy pictures

# chapter nine

# constitutional treatment and remedy types

Many people think that homoeopathy is only about helping colds get better or healing injuries after accidents. These uses represent just the tip of the iceberg.

When Samuel Hahnemann first started treating people with homoeopathy, he treated mostly acute diseases or the acute phase of a chronic disease. The patients usually improved, but the disease often came back. This disappointed Hahnemann, and he decided to investigate further. He wanted to find a way to treat the source that the acute disease sprang from. He focused his attention on how the patients were *between* acute attacks. The factors he observed acknowledged the person as a whole, and included such things as weather, food, sleeping habits, and their loves, fears, hates and general behaviour. He then decided to try to find a remedy that suited the person, not just the acute disease. What an amazing discovery when he found out that this approach worked! He called it *constitutional treatment.*

When we use a remedy for constitutional treatment we are treating chronic diseases. Some remedies are used primarily as constitutional remedies, but this does not mean that they cannot also be used for acute conditions.

Since Hahnemann developed this approach there have been further observations made by those homoeopaths who have followed in his footsteps. Out of this came the idea of remedy pictures or remedy types. The total nature or disposition of a person becomes in many instances more important than where in the body the disease is located. For example, if your child is weepy, demands affection and takes a dislike to hot stuffy rooms and rich foods, we would say he was a *Pulsatilla* type, because in the provings these are all symptoms of *Pulsatilla*. The constitutional treatment for this child would be to give him *Pulsatilla* regardless of his physical symptoms. By this method your child's total mental, emotional and physical state is taken into consideration. In this way we treat the sick child, not just the disease.

A homoeopath will put all this information together and try to find a remedy that will stimulate your child's innate healing capacity. We often find a link between the state of the mother during pregnancy, and that of her child. Both may actually need the same homoeopathic treatment. This is fascinating, as it shows us that the condition of the mother can influence the state of the developing foetus on many levels.

Constitutional treatment can be very profound and requires more knowledge of homoeopathy than is outlined in this book. For this reason, while we have included certain constitutional remedies in the **Materia Medica**, we have done so more for your information than for you to prescribe or use at home. Should you wish your child to receive constitutional treatment, consult a professional homoeopath.

## Constitutional Treatment for a Child with Recurrent Colds

A one-year-old boy has had 24 colds since he was born. He seems to be sick all the time, as he is only really well for three or four days a month.

### SYMPTOMS

colds, fever, vomiting
very sweet and friendly manner in the clinic
has had asthma and used a ventolin inhaler once
when he has a cold he sometimes vomits
can start off with a croup-cough, sometimes accompanied by rapid breathing
greenish-yellow discharge from his nose
very lethargic with the colds
used to be constipated, now stool tends to be black, almost tarry
has received many courses of antibiotics
wants to be held quite often, almost all the time when he is sick
clinging, whiny
loves to be outside; does not seem to be affected by cold weather
cries when his mother disappears; generally likes other people around, but
    when he is sick he just wants his mother
brings up his milk
sleep is restless and broken
is easily startled by loud noises

Based on his gentle, weepy, clinging temperament, along with his love of being outdoors, this baby was given *Pulsatilla 200*. After the first dose his cold cleared up and the constipation cleared up. His 'good periods' continued to lengthen as his general health improved.

As this example illustrates, a child's mental state or disposition is often the key to finding the best and most appropriate remedy.

chapter ten

# materia medica of important homoeopathic remedies

### Key

For each remedy in this Materia Medica we have provided a general description, often followed by information on four different aspects of the remedy:

1 Common Complaints: the illnesses or problems which the remedy helps best
2 Characteristic Symptoms: the signs that indicate which remedy is called for
3 Modalities: the situations/circumstances that can make the condition either better or worse
4 Typical Behaviour: the emotional symptoms, behavioural patterns and constitutional characteristics your child will display if she needs the remedy

(Where one or more of these aspects are not described, this is because the remedy is most useful in acute situations, so that information on modalities or typical behaviour is not applicable.)

In addition, where helpful we have provided further information about specific complaints for which a given remedy is useful – so, for example, under *Aconite* there are sections on Diarrhoea, Fever, Flu/Colds/Laryngitis/ Tonsillitis, and Nosebleeds – along with descriptions of each complaint's particular signs and symptoms.

## Aconite – Monkshood

*Aconite* is a very useful remedy at the onset of a sudden fever, and for complaints that arise after a shock or fright. The typical behaviour picture outlined below is extremely important, and must be present to some degree if using this remedy is to be a success.

### COMMON COMPLAINTS

◆ acute inflammations
◆ sudden pain
◆ onset of fever
◆ shock or fever accompanied by intense fear of death

### CHARACTERISTIC SYMPTOMS

1 Ailments such as a cough, cold, fever after exposure to cold.
2 Ailments after shock, with intense fears, particularly of death.
3 Any sudden ailments which are violent and painful.
4 Panic attacks that include restlessness, and fear of death or of pain.
5 Sufferer will be hot, dry and thirsty.

### MODALITIES

Worse for     severe cold weather, dry cold winds, night, being chilled
Better for    open air, rest

### TYPICAL BEHAVIOUR

Symptoms are intense and start very quickly when *Aconite* is indicated. Your child will be extremely fearful and restless, and may have a high fever. Older children may ask if they are going to die, or exhibit some other sign of a fear of death. They will be hot, dry and thirsty with a rapid pulse.

*Aconite* may also be useful in a situation where a child has been terrified, by either a real or imaginary event.

*Diarrhoea*

Particularly in infants, during the summer months, where the stools look green. May be accompanied by inflammation or fever.

*Fever*

*Aconite* helps with acute febrile conditions (fevers), whatever the diagnosis, providing at least one of the characteristic symptoms (listed above) is present.

- ◆ tremendous restlessness and great thirst.
- ◆ one cheek may be pale and cool while the other is flushed and hot
- ◆ your child may moan

*Flus, Colds, Laryngitis, Tonsillitis*

For the first stage of such ailments, if there is congestion, headaches and flushed skin. Severe sneezing, husky voice or laryngitis.

*Nose Bleeds*

Sudden nose bleed, accompanied by any of the above characteristic symptoms, would indicate *Aconite*.

## Apis mellifica – Bee venom

### COMMON COMPLAINTS

- ◆ insect bites
- ◆ hives
- ◆ allergic reactions
- ◆ throat and tonsil ailments

### CHARACTERISTIC SYMPTOMS

1  burning and stinging pains
2  no thirst

### MODALITIES

Worse for    hot air, hot applications, when in a warm bed, when touched

Better for    coolness, motion and open air

### TYPICAL BEHAVIOUR

Child will be irritable, restless, excitable and fidgety. She may exhibit a tendency towards jealousy. If feverish, she may go from an agitated state to one of apathy and exhaustion.

*Eyes*

Swollen, puffy lids. Styes. Stinging, bloodshot eyes.

*Skin*

This remedy can relieve many insect bites, especially bee stings. It can also help any rosy, inflamed spots on the skin where there is burning soreness and stinging and the skin looks or feels as if it might burst, it is so swollen. Usually the skin swellings are better for cool water and worse for warm applications.

*Throat and Tonsils*

Swollen, accompanied by stinging, burning pains.
The areas affected tend to be red or pink; symptoms improve if the child is given cool drinks, and are made worse if given warm drinks.

## Arnica montana – Leopard's bane

### COMMON COMPLAINTS

◆ head injuries
◆ bruises due to injuries
◆ black eye from injuries
◆ nosebleeds

### CHARACTERISTIC SYMPTOMS

1 bruised, lame, aching feeling caused by exertion, accident or a blow
2 passive bleeding due to injuries

### MODALITIES

Worse for      touch, motion, damp, cold
Better for      rest

### TYPICAL BEHAVIOUR

This is a great first-aid remedy. It is the number one remedy to think of in any injury where there is (or the possibility exists for) bruising. It will help deal with the shock of injuries. It is useful for children who are always banging themselves or falling out of trees or down the stairs. Along with the shock they often will say they do not need help and wish to be left alone.

## Arsenicum album

### COMMON COMPLAINTS

◆ gastrointestinal disorders such as diarrhoea
◆ traveller's diarrhoea
◆ food poisoning
◆ fevers
◆ colds

### CHARACTERISTIC SYMPTOMS

1 Burning pains, better for heat.
2 Child is thirsty for small sips of a drink.
3 Extreme restlessness and anxiety.
4 Child needs company.
5 Weakness, pallor.
6 Sensitivity to the cold.

### MODALITIES

Worse for     cold, night (particularly between midnight and
               3 a.m.)
Better for     heat, warm covers, warm applications, changing
               position

## TYPICAL BEHAVIOUR

When a child needing *Arsenicum* is ill she can be very demanding and tearful. She can be both restless and weak at the same time. This behaviour may seem out of proportion to the severity of the illness and can happen very rapidly. The child may be very fearful and can be very anxious about being left alone. She generally seems over-sensitive to everything. The child needing *Arsenicum* may also be very fastidious and controlling, demanding that everything be put in its proper place.

### Colds

A restless child with a head cold accompanied by sneezing, red eyes and nose and a profuse watery discharge which often reddens the area it runs over.

### Fever

Sudden great weakness accompanied by restlessness, irritability and anxiety. The child wants lots of attention, as she feels fearful. She may sip a warm drink, as cold drinks sometimes upset the stomach. She has chills with the fever.

### Gastroenteritis

Any gastric upset, particularly if you think it might be food poisoning. Vomiting and diarrhoea, sometimes simultaneously, or nausea accompanied by purging and watery stools. Cramping pains and great weakness with the diarrhoea.

## Aurum metallicum – Gold

The children who need *Aurum* are very introverted, as are those who need *Natrum muriaticum*. They do not show their emotions and are very quiet and serious. They are often isolated from their peer group because they are extremely bright. These children strive to come first in the class because they want to be the best and at the top of the school. They often look quite serious; their mothers will say that they need a lot of love and appreciation. They are so sensitive that any upset, shock or loss can result in their becoming even more reserved, depressed and melancholic.

If you find your child, after suffering some grief or loss, behaving in the ways we have described or which you find disturbing, please take her to see a professional homoeopath who can prescribe the correct treatment. Remedies such as *Natrum muriaticum* and *Aurum metallicum* can help your child come to terms with the changes in her life without becoming more chronically depressed.

## Baryta carbonica

### COMMON COMPLAINTS

◆ delayed development
◆ difficulty learning at school
◆ frequent colds accompanied by glandular swellings

### CHARACTERISTIC SYMPTOMS

This is usually used as a constitutional remedy and should be prescribed by a professional homoeopath. The indications for it are usually based on the typical behaviour outlined below. If you think your child may need *Baryta*, please do contact a qualified homoeopath.

### TYPICAL BEHAVIOUR

The child needing this remedy is often small and may look old beyond her years. Her body will show signs of difficulty assimilating food (she will be quite thin). It may also be indicated in a child who used to be fat but who has become emaciated, such as after vaccinations. There is considerable swelling of the glands, particularly the tonsils and adenoids, and the child may often talk through her nose. A child such as this is always a little bit behind and cannot learn easily. She tries very hard, but somehow the lessons just do not sink in. She is timid and shy and will stay very near to her mother. Her fears can be so great she may even hide behind her parents in the presence of strangers.

Her attachment to her parents is very deep and she often has anxieties and fears that something will happen to them. She generally hates school because of her attachment to family and her fears, as well as the fact that she does not understand the lessons and maybe the other children tease her. Such a child is often subjected to all sorts of tests, for physical problems or for mental slowness.

Homoeopaths have found that this remedy aids assimilation and that the child starts to thrive over a period of time both mentally and physically, catching up easily with her contemporaries.

The physical problems she suffers from are colds and swollen glands. This remedy may also be indicated for small or undeveloped genitals.

## Belladonna – Deadly nightshade

### COMMON COMPLAINTS

- fevers
- headaches
- influenza
- earache
- teething troubles
- swollen glands
- sore throats/tonsillitis

### CHARACTERISTIC SYMPTOMS

1 Sudden onset.
2 Dryness.
3 Intense throbbing pain accompanied by fullness or congestion.
4 Restlessness accompanied by twitching and spasms, maybe even delirium.
5 Very high fever accompanied by red face and dilated blood-shot eyes.
6 Redness of the inflamed part.
7 Desires lemonade.

### MODALITIES

Worse for    light, noise, jarring, draughts, being touched, having a hair-cut, heat of the sun

Better for    lying in bed, keeping still, darkness

#### TYPICAL BEHAVIOUR

Aggression in a normally well-behaved child. The problems start very rapidly. The fever is very intense. The child seems to radiate heat. She may sometimes want to bite or strike out at someone when not feeling well. *See* **Fever**, immediately below, for more details of the behaviour of a child needing *Belladonna*.

#### Ears

Sudden earache, particularly on the right-hand side. The child wakes out of sleep crying. The ear may be bright red and the pain throbbing.

#### Fever

The child's face is red hot; the pupils may be dilated. The skin on the body may be hot to the touch, though the hands and feet may be cold. Temperature can be as high as 39°C/104°F. If the child has a headache, she can complain that it feels like an intense throbbing. A normally well-behaved child when needing *Belladonna* for a fever might become aggressive and demanding, even biting and kicking. At other times the fever may produce nightmares, fears, hallucinations or delirium. The child may grind her teeth during sleep, and twitch and jerk her limbs. Although the thirst is not marked, the child will often crave lemonade or even wish to suck on a lemon.

#### Nose

Nosebleed, bright blood, starts suddenly; the child's face will be red.

#### Sore Throats

Including the early stages of tonsillitis where there is burning pain and possible loss of the voice. The throat becomes sore very rapidly and may be bright red. The soreness may be worse on the right-hand side.

*Teeth*

Teething problems where the child cries a lot, her face red hot or her gums extremely inflamed and painful.

## Bryonia – Wild hops

### COMMON COMPLAINTS

◆ flus and fevers
◆ digestive disorders
◆ respiratory problems

### CHARACTERISTIC SYMPTOMS

1 Dryness of all mucous membranes, including those along the digestive tract.
2 Constipation; stools are hard and dry.
3 All complaints worse for motion.
4 Thirst for large quantities; mouth and throat very dry.
5 Sharp, stitching pains.
6 Child wants to be left alone.

### MODALITIES

Worse for      movement of all kinds, being jarred, rising from a prone position, warm covers or a warm room, hot muggy weather, deep breathing (with respiratory problems)

Better for      pressure on painful area, cool air, cool water, a darkened room

### TYPICAL BEHAVIOUR

A child needing *Bryonia* in an acute crisis may appear very irritable and grumpy, wanting to be left alone. She will usually complain of dryness and is very thirsty for large amounts of water at infrequent intervals. She feels worse for any movement, whatever the main complaint is.

*Cough*

Dry, painful cough which sometimes forces the child to put her hands to her chest to hold it.

Chest may be painful from coughing or from deep breathing.

*Digestion*

Constipation with hard, dry stools.

There may be irritability with the constipation.

Diarrhoea worse in the morning after rising from bed and moving about.

Summer diarrhoea, especially after getting hot and then having a cold drink.

*Fevers*

The fever that calls for *Bryonia* develops slowly, usually during damp weather or sometimes when the weather turns from cold to warm. The child may have a pressure headache that is worse for the slightest movement. Possible dizziness when getting up from lying down. Dry mouth, at times coated (with a white tongue). Great thirst for water accompanies the fever.

*Head*

Headaches worse for motion, even the movement of the eyes.

Worse for coughing.

Often left-sided.

*Measles*

*Bryonia* is useful when the eruptions are slow to come out or they come out and then recede and your child gets worse again.

## Calcarea carbonica

### COMMON COMPLAINTS

This is primarily used as a constitutional remedy for slowness of development and problems with metabolism, assimilation and elimination. These can include glandular, skin, digestive and respiratory disorders.

It should only be prescribed by a professional homoeopath.

### CHARACTERISTIC SYMPTOMS

1 Head sweats easily, especially in bed.
2 Flabbiness, obesity.
3 Teeth and bones slow to develop.
4 Walking and talking may be delayed.
5 Sourness of discharges.
6 Poor stamina.
7 Child craves eggs.
8 Suffers from a variety of fears and anxieties.

### MODALITIES

Worse for     cold wet weather, exertion, during teething, milk
Better for    dry weather

### TYPICAL BEHAVIOUR (INCLUDING METABOLIC PROBLEMS)

This is a common remedy and is particularly useful in children whose development is delayed in some way (slow to walk, talk or develop teeth). We also find that these children can have low resistance to infections, swollen glands, colds, earaches and chest infections.

They are generally very cheerful, affectionate and easy-going with people they know. They are frequently on the plumpish side, with rosy red cheeks. In some cases they can develop problems with milk tolerance, in which case they may be underweight.

They lack stamina and do not play as actively as other children. They tend to watch other children play, and can be a little reserved and withdrawn. This reserved nature is also noticeable when they are with strangers, until they get to know them.

We would also consider this remedy for anxious children who may have a curiosity about God but fears of the dark, the devil, death, dogs and mice.

Children who need *Calcarea carbonica* as a constitutional remedy perspire very easily, especially around the head. This is noticeable when they exert themselves in any way, or when they go to bed at night.

They often love their food, including all forms of carbohydrates particularly sugar, cakes and biscuits. Eggs are another favourite. You may also notice them sucking on indigestible things such as pencils or rubbers, or eating mud or sand from the garden. When they get to school age they can be very studious, but again (like those needing *Baryta carbonica*) they find it difficult to understand and assimilate what they are being taught.

## Cantharis

### COMMON COMPLAINTS

◆ burns (including sunburn)
◆ cystitis

### CHARACTERISTIC SYMPTOMS

1 Pain is violent, cutting and burning.
2 Burned skin forms blisters very quickly.
3 With cystitis, there is burning and cutting pain, an intolerable urge to urinate but passing of only a few drops at a time.

### MODALITIES

Worse for      touch
Better for      warmth, rest, cold applications

## Chamomilla

### COMMON COMPLAINTS

◆ teething problems
◆ fevers
◆ diarrhoea/colic
◆ earaches
◆ difficult, irritable behaviour

### CHARACTERISTIC SYMPTOMS

1 Intolerable pain accompanied by excessive irritability.
2 Nothing satisfies the child.
3 Feels better only when being carried.
4 Offensive stool.

### MODALITIES

Worse for       teething, anger, cold air, 9 p.m. to midnight
Better for      being carried

### TYPICAL BEHAVIOUR

Children needing *Chamomilla* are very irritable, peevish and restless. They are highly sensitive to the slightest pain or interference. They may get angry if you so much as even glance at them. They can sometimes be snappish and fretful. Nothing can satisfy them, they want things, then throw them away demanding something else. They can sometimes be quite aggressive, hitting out and striking others. In acute situations they can be so demanding that their parents may have to carry them all the time just to keep them calm, as they can become quite inconsolable. If they hurt themselves or are in pain, they seem abnormally sensitive and scream because they cannot bear even a relatively minor problem.

*Diarrhoea/colic*
Offensive stools that can sometimes smell like rotten eggs and look like 'chopped eggs and spinach'.

This diarrhoea and sometimes extremely painful colic often accompany teething, making the child very irritable and inconsolable. The colic may cause her to arch her back.

*Earache*

An important remedy for middle ear inflammations which are worse at night and accompanied by irritability. The child can sometimes become almost hysterical.

*Teething*

*Chamomilla* is frequently indicated when a child is teething. Your child will be very irritable at this time and, depending on which tooth is erupting, one cheek can be red and the other pale.

## Ferrum phosphoricum

### COMMON COMPLAINTS

◆ earaches
◆ sore throats
◆ fevers
◆ chest complaints

### CHARACTERISTIC SYMPTOMS

1  Low-grade fever.
2  Flushing of the face; there may be red circles on the cheeks.
3  General body ache.
4  Weakness.
5  Child may be subject to haemorrhage, such as a nosebleed.
6  Useful when the symptoms first show.

### MODALITIES

Worse for      night, motion, being jarred, cold air
Better for      lying down

*Fevers*

Early stages of a fever when there are no other clear behavioural indications such as we have mentioned for other remedies. This remedy can be for nondescript fevers which do not seem to cause problems anywhere else in the body, or when they localize in the throat, ear or chest. The child will not be restless (as she would if she needed *Aconite* or *Belladonna*), nor will she be completely worn out (as when she needs *Gelsemium*). She will be somewhere between these two states. The low-grade fever may be accompanied by a nosebleed; your child's face may be either flushed or pale.

## Gelsemium – Yellow jasmine

### COMMON COMPLAINTS

◆ influenza and colds that come on slowly
◆ exam nerves

### CHARACTERISTIC SYMPTOMS

1 Weariness, general weakness and dizziness.
2 Sleepiness accompanied by a dull, dopey feeling.
3 Stiffness accompanied by heaviness in the body and legs.
4 Child does not want to be bothered.
5 No thirst, even though feverish.

### MODALITIES

Worse for       spring; humid, foggy, cold, damp weather; sun; summer heat; muggy, heavy weather; ordeals such as exams; fright; bad news; shock

Better for      sweating

### TYPICAL BEHAVIOUR

The child will be apprehensive in response to new situations or ordeals such as exams. This can lead to trembling and weakness. With flu, the child can often be so weak that she wants to be left alone. It is as if she has no energy for anything at all.

### *Anticipation of Ordeals*

This can be exams, after receiving bad news, or any situation that brings on anxiety, weakness and trembling and often an attack of diarrhoea along with it.

*Fevers*

Overpowering drowsiness, dullness and aching. Can be accompanied by dizziness and trembling. The eyelids seem heavy and drooping; the child may have a headache as well. She seems withdrawn and may even be expressionless, she is feeling so unwell. She may complain of chills running up and down the spine; her lack of thirst is noticeable.

*Head*

Headaches from exposure to the sun that cause a sense of congestion along with dullness, heaviness and drowsiness. Pain at the back of the head.

## Hepar sulphuris

### COMMON COMPLAINTS

- respiratory conditions – laryngitis, bronchitis, pleurisy, pneumonia
- ear complaints
- glandular swellings, tonsillitis, sore throats
- wounds that are slow to heal – boils, abscesses, infected cuts, etc.

### CHARACTERISTIC SYMPTOMS

1 Hypersensitivity of the nervous system.
2 Child is extremely chilly.
3 Sour or offensive discharges and secretions.
4 Irritability accompanied by possibly violent impulses.
5 Stitch-like or splinter-like pains.
6 Tendency to pus formation.
7 Extremely painful abscesses.
8 Painful parts very sensitive to touch and cold.

### MODALITIES

Worse for     cold dry wind, cold air, cold draughts, cold food and drink, touch, night

Better for     warmth, after eating, damp weather

**TYPICAL BEHAVIOUR**

Very irritable, abusive and impatient. Sensitive to the slightest criticism, slightest touch, draught, slightest exposure to cold or noise. The oversensitivity may cause violent outbursts. Violent dreams, possibly of fire.

*Ears*

Inflammation of the middle ear (otitis media).

Child wakes screaming in the night and the ear cannot be touched.

The ear is very sensitive to the slightest degree of cold air. (*See also* **Belladonna** and **Chamomilla**)

Often better for warm applications.

Glands around the neck or under the ear may be swollen.

*Skin*

Boils, abscesses and whitlows that are extremely painful to touch and improved by heat.

*Throat, Chest and Coughs*

Inflammation of the throat and/or tonsils.

Pain feels like splinters or broken glass, or as if something is stuck in the throat.

Tonsils swollen, may have pus on them.

Pain better for warm drinks.

Croupy cough, worse at night and after exposure to cold.

Barking cough may be accompanied by night sweats.

Swollen glands.

Respiratory problems.

## Hypericum – St John's Wort

### COMMON COMPLAINTS

- injuries to places where there are nerve endings, such as the tips of fingers or toes or the base of the spine
- puncture wounds
- insect bites and animal bites
- back pains

### CHARACTERISTIC SYMPTOMS

1 Any puncture wounds caused by sharp objects such as nails or splinters; insect stings, animal bites and scratches accompanied by swelling and inflammation.
2 Shooting pains; pains may shoot along the pathway of a nerve up the limb where the injury took place.
3 Nerve pain in the gums after dental extractions or deep drilling.
4 Crushed fingertips or toes after an accident.
5 Injury to coccyx (base of spine).
6 Shooting pains down the arm after nerve injury to the neck area.

This is one of the great first-aid remedies used in homoeopathy. It helps heal wounded or bruised nerves. Where there is an injury to the tips of fingers or toes, it will quickly help relieve the pain and, where necessary, assist in the growth of new nails. This remedy alone has convinced many people of the value of homoeopathy in first-aid situations.

## Ipecacuanha

### COMMON COMPLAINTS

◆ digestive disorders – nausea, diarrhoea
◆ respiratory problems – coughs, bronchitis
◆ nosebleeds

### CHARACTERISTIC SYMPTOMS

1 Persistent nausea and vomiting, sometimes accompanied by profuse salivation.
2 Nausea that is not relieved by vomiting.
3 Clean or pink tongue where you would expect a coated tongue.
4 No thirst.
5 Haemorrhages of bright red blood, such as nosebleeds, sometimes accompanied by nausea.

Persistent nausea that is not relieved by anything whatsoever is a chief characteristic symptom of *Ipecacuanha*. This nausea may be present when there are other symptoms such as respiratory problems.

### MODALITIES

Worse for  warmth, warm damp weather, being in a warm room, overeating – pork, veal, rich foods, ice-cream; the smell of food, cold nights after hot days

Better for  open air

### TYPICAL BEHAVIOUR

The child is irritable, impatient, restless and does not know what she wants. Complaints may start after being punished.
The face may be pale, the eyes sunken.

*Chest and Respiratory Problems*
Whooping cough, bronchitis, children's coughs often accompanied by rattling and wheezing in the chest.
Chest seems full of mucus, which is difficult to cough up.
Suffocative cough accompanied by retching and vomiting.
The child ends up gagging and choking and may become blue.
Nausea and/or vomiting can accompany these coughs.

*Digestive Disorders*

Nausea is constant and nothing helps it.

Often after rich foods such as ice-cream, pork or pastry.

Nausea and vomiting accompanied by headaches, haemorrhages, coughs.

Possibly grassy green, slimy stools.

*Nose*

Nosebleeds of bright red blood accompanied by coughs or whooping cough.

Nosebleeds accompanied by the mental state outlined above, or by nausea.

## Ledum

### COMMON COMPLAINTS

- ◆ puncture wounds
- ◆ animal bites, insect stings
- ◆ bruises/swelling, black eyes
- ◆ damage to the eyes, fibrous tissue, joints, tendons, periosteum

### CHARACTERISTIC SYMPTOMS

1 wounded areas are cold to the touch
2 long-lasting discolouration after injuries, black or blue marks turning green
3 a lot of swelling and inflammation after a bite or sting

### MODALITIES

Worse for    warmth, motion

Better for    cold applications, cold air, rest, eating (counteracts any accompanying headache)

## Lycopodium – Club moss

### COMMON COMPLAINTS

- ◆ colic in babies, digestive disorders and gastric upsets
- ◆ sore throats
- ◆ tonsillitis
- ◆ bronchitis and other respiratory complaints

### CHARACTERISTIC SYMPTOMS

1 Craves sugar/sweets.
2 Intolerant of starches.
3 Bloating, flatulence.
4 Right-sided complaints or complaints that travel from the right to left side.
5 Headaches after indigestion.
6 Intense hunger, but feels full after a few mouthfuls.
7 All complaints may be worse between 4 and 8 p.m.

### MODALITIES

Worse for     4 to 8 p.m., heat, being contradicted, 'flatulent' foods (i.e., foods that produce wind)

Better for     warm drinks, motion, loosening clothing

### TYPICAL BEHAVIOUR

These children may feel anxious in new situations. Babies sometimes are noticeably apprehensive with strangers and may frown as their way of expressing this apprehension. In older children, visiting a friend's house for the first time might make the child feel very insecure, but should the friends come to the child's house her behaviour can be noticeably bossy rather than anxious. In other words, the child can be domineering when she feels secure and timid and cowardly when she feels less sure of herself and her surroundings.

Children who need this remedy are also quite anxious about strangers, hate to be left alone and are afraid of the dark. When they get older their fears may centre more around monsters and ghosts; at school they will be very sensitive to being teased and having to speak up in front of the class. Their fears and anxieties can bring about physical symptoms such as tummy ache and diarrhoea or constipation.

Babies who need *Lycopodium* often have colic; in older children we have found that overeating, particularly of sweets, may produce headaches, severe indigestion and wind.

These children are also prone to skin conditions e.g. eczema.

This remedy is used for acute complaints but is also very frequently helpful as a deep-acting constitutional remedy.

### Digestion
Repeated digestive disorders including colic.
Acidity, bloating and flatulence after even a small amount of food.
May fill up quickly on eating; needs to loosen her clothes around the waist, especially if bloated.

### Head
Pains worse on the right side, or which travel from the right to the left side.
Headaches from overeating.

### Throat and Tonsil Problems
Problems often start first on the right side and may move to the left. Usually the throat pains may be eased by warm drinks, though occasionally also by cold drinks.

## Mercurius vivus

#### COMMON COMPLAINTS
◆ earache
◆ flus and fevers
◆ mumps
◆ tonsillitis

#### CHARACTERISTIC SYMPTOMS
1 Foul-smelling breath.
2 Increased salivation, particularly at night.
3 Sweating that does not relieve the condition.
4 Intense thirst.
5 Trembling, such as during fever.
6 Sensitivity to heat and cold.
7 Swollen glands.
8 Burning pains.

**MODALITIES**

Worse for       night, changes in the outside temperature,
                aggravation, perspiration

Better for      moderate temperatures, rest, morning

**TYPICAL BEHAVIOUR**

The child needing this remedy may be irritable, complaining, discontented and oversensitive.

### Digestion

Intense thirst for cold drinks. Craves bread and butter. Diarrhoea will be offensive. The child may feel that she constantly needs to pass a stool.

### Ears

Pain worse at night and accompanied by a thick yellow or blood-streaked discharge from the ear. Swollen glands.

### Face

Mouth ulcers accompanied by offensive breath and increased salivation.

### Fevers

Profuse perspiration that does not deliver relief. Alternating chills and fever. Child becomes overheated easily by the warmth of her bed.

### Sore Throats and Tonsillitis

Burning in the throat. Swollen glands accompanied by severe pain on swallowing. Offensive breath accompanied by salivation; there may be ulcers on the tonsils.

## Natrum muriaticum – Sodium chloride

### COMMON COMPLAINTS

◆ catarrh
◆ cold sores on the mouth
◆ headaches in school children, especially girls
◆ problems after grief

### CHARACTERISTIC SYMPTOMS

1 Desire for salty food, thirst.
2 Worse for the heat of the sun.
3 Better or worse for the seaside.
4 Discharge that resembles egg-whites.
5 Child seems emotionally 'closed'.

### MODALITIES

Worse for    being consoled, intellectual work, heat of the sun,
            10 a.m., being at the seaside
Better for   fresh open air, sweating, being at the seaside

The child can be better or worse by the sea.

### TYPICAL BEHAVIOUR

Children needing *Natrum muriaticum* are generally introverted and quiet. They often like to be alone and are very sensitive to others' feelings. If upset they will often disappear into their bedroom and cry alone rather than show their feelings in public. Sometimes mothers of such children describe their children as seemingly cool and distant on the outside but craving lots of love and affection underneath. They are not exactly anxious children, but shocks or family problems such as divorce, death or loss may leave them in a state of hysteria to be followed by greater introversion.

As they get older and go to school, you may notice that these children do not make friends easily but concentrate hard on their studies and are very serious. In groups or at parties they will often stand to one side, watching the other children play or interact.

They tend to like sad, melancholy music.

They also like to be quite alone while they read, often taking themselves off to their room or to a quiet corner where they will not be disturbed at all.

*Natrum muriaticum* is useful for both acute and chronic disorders.

*Face*

Mouth ulcers on gums, tongue or inside mouth.

Cracks on lips or around the corners of the mouth.

Cold sores on the lips or face.

Cold sores after exposure to the sun.

*Head*

Headaches after grief/upset, studying too much.

Worse for exposure to the sun.

Worse for noise, light, reading.

Throbbing headaches like many little hammers knocking on the brain.

*Nose*

Hay fever, catarrh with a raw egg-white-like discharge.

Sneezing that precedes a cold.

Cold or hay fever that is accompanied by a loss of smell or taste.

*Sleep*

Insomnia after grief.

## Nux vomica – Poison nut

### COMMON COMPLAINTS

◆ stomach disorders
◆ flu and fevers
◆ constipation

### CHARACTERISTIC SYMPTOMS

1 Child is often very chilly.
2 Constipation, though child still feels urgency even after she has been to the toilet.
3 Constipation when travelling.
4 Irritability and impatience.
5 Oversensitivity to noise, smells, criticism, etc.
6 Desire for strong-tasting foods.
7 Cramps.
8 Indigestion brought on by overeating.

### MODALITIES

Worse for      morning, cold air, after eating
Better for     warmth, rest, loosening clothes around the waist (if indigestion is the problem)

### TYPICAL BEHAVIOUR

Children who need *Nux vomica* often suffer from digestive problems and are irritable. They hate criticism and can be bossy, rude, ambitious and competitive. They can often be hard workers, and become quite upset if they do not do well at school.

*Colds*

Child will be easily irritated and will ask to be kept warm at all times. For infant snuffles. They may have a dry stuffed-up nose at night, but it runs during the day.

*Digestive Tract*

Lack of appetite. Nausea, indigestion or cramping shortly after eating. Child may also feel nauseated or may actually vomit in the morning. With the nausea she may feel that if she could only vomit she would feel better. Constipation accompanied by a continuous urging for stool, but whenever she does pass stool it can feel as if something is still left behind.

*Fevers and Flu*

Often accompanied by irritability and a desire to lie completely still under the covers. The slightest little movement makes the child feel chilly.

*Head*

Pain from overeating or with constipation.

## Phosphorus

### COMMON COMPLAINTS

♦ colds
♦ nosebleeds
♦ anxieties
♦ respiratory/chest infections
♦ hypersensitivity
♦ digestive complaints

### CHARACTERISTIC SYMPTOMS

1  Tendency to bleed easily from any wound.
2  Rapid growth.
3  Burning pains.
4  Congestion sometimes accompanied by blood-streaked discharges.
5  Child craves salt, savoury foods, ice-cold drinks and ice-cream.
6  Thirst.
7  Desire to eat at night.
8  Child is extremely sensitive, open and impressionable.
9  Sympathetic and affectionate; likes people.
10  Fearful and nervous.

### MODALITIES
Worse for    cold weather, emotional upsets, lying on painful side, thunderstorms, sudden weather changes

Better for    being rubbed or massaged, eating, catnaps or sleep

### TYPICAL BEHAVIOUR
Children needing *Phosphorus* are warm and affectionate. They easily make contact, even with strangers. They are extremely sympathetic, especially if someone is unwell. With this sensitivity they can suffer badly from emotional upsets.

They are often slender with fine hair and eyelashes. Their fingers are long, thin and delicate; their skin is often like white porcelain. At school they may do well in the more artistic lessons. They are very excitable and have a strong imagination, but sometimes this means that they suffer badly from fears.

Their anxieties can be non-specific or, in more extreme cases, their vivid imagination makes them very scared of the dark. They can imagine their clothes on the chair in the bedroom turning into ghosts or evil witches.

They can start asking questions about death and disease and can be very anxious if they are ill, especially if left alone. Cuddles, touching and reassurance help them feel less anxious when they are sick.

*Phosphorus* is used as both a constitutional and an acute remedy.

#### Digestion
Very thirsty for cold drinks.

Likes ice-cream, salt, fizzy drinks, chocolate.

Burning pains in stomach.

Digestive problems (accompanied by nausea and sometimes vomiting) that are better for cold drinks – though the child may vomit after a cold drink warms up in her stomach.

Diarrhoea which may be eased by cold drinks.

Anus feels wide open; the stool is involuntary, and watery or thin.

#### Nose
Nosebleeds of bright red blood in children with the type of character traits outlined above.

*Respiratory Complaints, Colds, Fevers*
Children who easily catch colds that go to the chest.

Tickling coughs that are worse when laughing, talking, if exposed to cold air, change of temperature, lying on the left side; better for sitting up.

Chest complaints with fever, breathlessness, painful cough, and sometimes blood-streaked expectoration.

Laryngitis accompanied by the modalities and typical behaviour of *Phosphorus.*

## Pulsatilla – Wind Flower

This is a very commonly used remedy for a variety of children's complaints, both acute and chronic. The prescription is usually made based on looking at the modalities, characteristic symptoms and especially the typical behaviour pattern. The typical behaviour picture in particular is extremely important when deciding whether or not to prescribe *Pulsatilla.* While with adults it is more commonly indicated for women than men, with children it is of equal use for either sex.

### COMMON COMPLAINTS

- earaches
- eye complaints
- colds, flus and fevers
- digestive complaints
- loneliness and clinginess
- measles
- mumps
- chicken pox

### CHARACTERISTIC SYMPTOMS

1  Yellow-green, thick, bland catarrh or discharges.
2  Wandering pains.
3  Lack of thirst, even during fever.
4  Worse in warm stuffy rooms or hot weather; better for open air.
5  Child is sensitive, weepy, emotional, changeable, moody; craves affection and sympathy.
6  Worse for eating fat or rich food.

## MODALITIES

Worse for    warm air, warm food and drinks, fatty or rich foods
(pork, ice-cream)

Better for   cool open air, consolation and sympathy, crying,
lying with head high or sitting semi-erect, cool
drinks, slowly walking about (especially in open air)

## TYPICAL BEHAVIOUR

This remedy is made from the Wind Flower; the name of the plant
suggests variability and vulnerability, and that is just how children
who need *Pulsatilla* are. They are extremely affectionate and lovable
one minute and can be in a bad mood the next. They weep easily and
can seem shy, then suddenly the next minute they are playful and
noisy. They can get terribly upset if they are criticized, and in general
feel much better after a good cry.

They are fearful of being alone and can develop symptoms if they
feel abandoned. They are extremely anxious and clingy, often asking
their parents 'Do you love me?' Due to this insecurity they are very
anxious to please. They may cry if they do not get attention, and
some mothers report that they are like little shadows that follow them
around all the time. They may also be afraid of the dark and of
ghosts.

It is worth mentioning here that *Pulsatilla* is a very good remedy
for young girls reaching puberty, when they are going through the
tremendous emotional upsets that can occur around the time of
menstruation – particularly if their periods are delayed or heavy.

They tend to do well in the fresh open air, but do not like to get
cold.

Their physical symptoms can be as changeable as their moods.
Their bowel movements may be different every day, and any pain can
travel from one part of the body to another.

*Digestion*

No thirst.

Child craves butter, ice-cream and cold foods. Fats and ice-cream can, however, aggravate the symptoms.

Indigestion, nausea, diarrhoea after eating rich foods, fats, pork or indigestion, accompanied by typical *Pulsatilla* behaviour.

*Earaches*

Otitis media affecting weepy children who crave comfort and sympathy.

Ear pain that is worse for heat and at night.

There may be greenish-yellow discharge from the ear.

*Eyes*

Conjunctivitis accompanied by a green or yellow discharge; better for cool applications.

*Fevers*

No thirst.

Child throws blankets off because of her aversion to heat.

*Measles, Mumps and Chicken Pox*

*See* relevant section (*pages 125, 127, 121*).

*Nose*

Profuse bland nasal discharge, greenish in colour.

Hay fever worse in warm rooms.

*Respiratory Complaints*

Cough at night that causes the child to sit up. Bronchitis.

Allergic asthma accompanied by the typical behaviour and modalities of *Pulsatilla.*

Difficult breathing that is worse at night, when lying flat, in a warm room, when feeling emotional.

Difficult breathing better for sitting up and open air, sometimes better for slowly walking about in the open air.

## Rhus toxicodendron – Poison Ivy

### COMMON COMPLAINTS

◆ soft-tissue injuries
◆ strains and sprains of muscles and tendons
◆ hives
◆ respiratory problems
◆ cold sores
◆ chicken pox

### CHARACTERISTIC SYMPTOMS

1 Symptoms better for continued motion.
2 Symptoms worse after resting for a while, for example first thing in morning, and when first getting up or stirring after being seated.
3 Child is very restless, tosses, turns, cannot keep still.

### MODALITIES

Worse for    resting and on first beginning to move; night, exposure to cold wet weather, getting wet (especially after being overheated), sprains, overexertion

Better for    heat, hot weather, slow continual motion of the entire body or affected part, changing position

### TYPICAL BEHAVIOUR

The child who needs *Rhus toxicodendron* is extremely restless and finds it hard to keep still. She is on the move constantly during the day and tosses and turns while in bed at night. She may be irritable, hurried and impatient.

The modalities and characteristic symptoms of *Rhus toxicodendron* are generally enough to provide us with a clear indication that it is the correct remedy to use.

*Face*

Cold sores around the lips; often worse for cold damp weather.
Cracks on corners of mouth.

*Respiratory Complaints*

Tickling coughs; worse for exposure to cold and damp.
Asthma, bronchitis that is worse for cold and damp; child is restless but feels worse after any exertion.
Chest complaints that arise from the suppression of the symptoms of eczema.

*Skin*

Hives or itching skin eruptions, better for very hot water.
For chicken pox which causes restlessness and is very itchy, especially at night.

*Sprains and Strains*

Sprains and strains caused by overexertion; for injuries that feel worse if the child tries to move after being at rest; better for continued motion – may only be eased if the child continually changes the position of the affected limb.

## Ruta graveolens – Rue

A useful first-aid remedy for aches, sprains and strains especially to the parts of the body listed below.

### COMMON COMPLAINTS

◆ injuries to the cartilages, tendons, outer covering of bones (periosteum) and ligaments
◆ injuries to wrist
◆ symptoms that arise after dental surgery

### CHARACTERISTIC SYMPTOMS

1 Tendons (especially in the knees and elbows) are painful after a strain.
2 Bruising to bones after injury.
3 Joint strains (when *Arnica* has been tried but is no longer helping).
4 Bruising to muscles (when *Arnica* or *Rhus toxicodendron* does not help).
5 Eye strain, possibly accompanied by headaches brought on by studying or delicate work such as drawing.
6 Small hard lumps (ganglia) that form after an injury to, for example, the wrist.
7 Useful after having a tooth removed, for pain that lingers even after *Arnica* has been given.

### MODALITIES

Worse for     over-exertion, cold and wet weather, pressure on the area

Better for     warmth

## Silica

### COMMON COMPLAINTS

◆ ear problems
◆ frequent colds and glandular problems
◆ constipation
◆ slowness of development and failure to thrive
◆ abscesses and wounds that are slow to heal

*Silica* is usually prescribed as a constitutional remedy. It has a profound affect on the metabolism and should only be prescribed by a professional homoeopath.

## CHARACTERISTIC SYMPTOMS

1 Offensive foot sweats.
2 Child is mild and apprehensive, with a yielding temperament and lacking in self-confidence.
3 Sensitivity to draughts and cold.
4 Brittle nails, thin hair.
5 Child is low in physical energy and drive.

### MODALITIES

Worse for     cold air, draughts, damp, milk, blocked perspiration (if your child's feet are sweaty you should not try to 'correct' this, as this will make her symptoms worse)

Better for     warmth

### TYPICAL BEHAVIOUR

The typical description of children needing *Silica* is that they 'lack grit'. They may lack stamina (physically, emotionally or mentally). They will often be well behaved, quiet, polite, hard-working pupils at school. They can also have a fear of failure.

They may be shy, apprehensive and fearful of new situations, such as appearing in front of the class or meeting strangers. You may notice that such children seem to give in easily during a quarrel; they keep their opinions to themselves and do not challenge others.

They often do not thrive well: as babies they can be weak and sickly, and may frequently bring up their milk. As young children they get repeated colds, enlarged tonsils, earaches and chest infections. The central precept of *Silica* is that children who need it seem to have some kind of metabolic problem which results in difficulty with food absorption, and which therefore leads to weight loss. Often accompanying this is thin hair, brittle nails and even problems with the bones.

Sometimes these children feel quite chilly a lot of the time, particularly when their glands are swollen. This is unusual, as most children are generally warm unless they are suffering from some kind of acute illness.

## Staphysagria – Stavesacre

### COMMON COMPLAINTS

◆ glandular swellings
◆ bedwetting
◆ bladder problems
◆ incised wounds (after surgery)
◆ skin problems

This is a remedy that we have found has helped children who are extremely sensitive from a very early age and are often introverted. It is usually prescribed constitutionally, based on observations of the child's typical behaviour.

Children who need *Staphysagria* take things very much to heart and can get upset and cry after the slightest reprimand. They can weep easily, though they usually tend to suppress their feelings. The exception to this will be the occasional outburst of anger and indignation, during which they will throw things.

Their anxiety may show itself in the form of bedwetting. This often happens when they are under stress, for example if they are being bullied at school. In other cases the anxiety may show itself in the development of skin problems.

If a child has a history of being teased, humiliated, involved in quarrels or exposed to any other kind of upset, in addition to suffering from a more obvious physical problem, a homoeopath might consider this remedy to help to ease the child's troubles.

Physically, any areas that are sore are worse for the least touch may indicate *Staphysagria*. In a sense, a child needing *Staphysagria* does not like to be 'touched' (physically or emotionally) wherever she feels most vulnerable.

## Sulphur

### COMMON COMPLAINTS

◆ anxieties
◆ skin complaints
◆ digestive disorders
◆ respiratory problems

### CHARACTERISTIC SYMPTOMS

1 Burning pains.
2 Unhealthy skin that is itchy (as in the case of allergy or eczema).
3 Wounds that are slow to heal.
4 Itching worse in warm bed at night.
5 Aversion to bathing.
6 Insomnia.
7 Diarrhoea.
8 Offensive discharges, sweat and stools.
9 Craves sugar, sweets and fatty foods.
10 Child may ask to have a sip of your beer or wine.
11 Aversion to heat, may throw blankets off during sleep.
12 Orifices of the body (such as ears, lips, anus) are often red.
13 Tendency to relapse.

### MODALITIES

Worse for     around 11 a.m., often accompanied by hunger;
              bathing, heat of the bed, heat in general, woollens,
              standing, weather changes
Better for    dry weather, open air

### TYPICAL BEHAVIOUR

Children who can benefit from *Sulphur* are often noticed to be extroverted from an early age. They are generally curious about everything. Even as toddlers they easily make friends with everyone. In a playground they will immediately run off to play with other children without any anxiety about the new situation. In a stranger's house they may want to investigate everything.

They are strong little characters and can be very determined (even bossy) about what they do or do not want. At school they can be very bright or very lazy; even the lazy ones will often have bright minds. At home they remain quite keen always to be reading a new book or investigating some intellectual problem. Both the laziness and the over-concern with books may show up as excessive untidiness and a lack of interest in anything else. They could be the type of children who get a school report saying 'bright child, but could do better'.

Children needing *Sulphur* reveal their anxiety in the form of worrying about their parents' safety. They get so anxious that they may dread leaving their parents when it's time to go to school. They may even come home from school at midday to make sure their parents are safe. Other noticeable worries are fear of ghosts, of robbers and poverty; they also may be frightened of lifts or heights.

These children get dirty more easily than other children and are not keen on washing themselves. Trying to get them to bed at night is almost impossible; they will always want to stay up with you. Their appetites are good but they often suffer from eczema or other skin complaints. Most skin complaints should be treated constitutionally by a professional homoeopath. *Sulphur* is also often used for chronic complaints.

*Rectum*

Red anus
Nappy rash
Anus itchy at night, especially when warm
Diarrhoea early in the morning (often wakes the child up)
Offensive stools

*Skin*

Itchy skin eruptions that are worse for wool, heat of the bed, bathing, night and warmth in general.

Recurrent boils and wounds that are slow to heal.

*Sulphur* is useful for all types of skin problems. The best prescriptions are made by careful observation of the modalities and typical behaviour of the child. Consult a homoeopath for chronic skin diseases such as eczema.

*Stomach*

Huge appetite, either for food or drinks. Aversion to eggs, especially the yolk

Heartburn, indigestion

Likes cold drinks

## Symphytum – Comfrey

### COMMON COMPLAINTS

◆ bone injuries
◆ fractures that are slow to knit
◆ eye injuries
◆ any trauma to the bones or the periosteum (the membrane over the surface of the bones)
◆ trauma to the eye after being damaged by a blunt weapon, such as a ball or a fist

## Urtica urens

### COMMON COMPLAINTS

◆ insect bites
◆ stings
◆ allergic skin reactions
◆ burns
◆ urticaria (nettle rash)
◆ the ill effects of eating shellfish
◆ after a first-degree burn (especially if caused by hot water) when there is a burning sensation and violent itching

### CHARACTERISTIC SYMPTOMS

1 After bites or stings where the skin itches, stings and burns (as with nettle rash or hives) and is eased by rubbing.
2 Severe swelling of a large area around the sting.

### MODALITIES

Worse for  cool air, cool applications
Better for  warmth

# glossary

**Causation** There can be a direct cause of an illness, such as a bump on the head or exposure to a wet, cold day; or an indirect cause, such as living in a stressful situation or being bullied at school

**Classical Homoeopathy** Homoeopaths use carefully selected remedies made from natural substances to stimulate a patient's vitality or immune system. The classical homoeopath gives only one remedy at a time. This remedy is chosen for the individual and is based on the totality of symptoms, including the mental, emotional and physical symptoms.

**Disease** An imbalance in the body's defences which produces changes in the sensations and the functioning on a mental, emotional and physical level. These signs and symptoms are Nature's warning of trouble within, and should not be suppressed.

**Disease, Acute** An acute disease has a distinct beginning and end. It usually runs through a limited course, characterized by three clear stages: the *prodromal* period, when symptoms are developing; the *acute* stage, when symptoms are fully present and there is the possibility of a fever; and the *convalescence* phase, when the sufferer recovers. Examples of acute illnesses include measles, flu, and pneumonia.

**Disease, Chronic** Chronic ailments are not self-limiting but can instead persist throughout a person's life (an earache that keeps coming back is an example). These recurrences (acute episodes) are a manifestation of a weakness in the immune system and need constitutional treatment.

**Health** Not just a state of being free from pain or discomfort on a physical level, but an ability to be creative and to adapt to changes and challenges that occur in life. Health is a state of harmony and a sense of well-being.

**Law of Similars** Based on the principle that any substance that is capable of causing symptoms in a healthy person also has the potential for healing those symptoms in a sick person if given in a small enough dose.

**Materia Medica** Books containing all relevant information needed about certain homoeopathic remedies.

**Modalities** Circumstances or things that make a person's symptoms either better or worse; examples might include heat, cold, motion, rest, pressure, foods, drinks.

**Polychrest** One of a group of remedies in the Materia Medica that have been shown to be of considerable help in a variety of different illnesses and which are therefore commonly prescribed.

**Potency** The strength of a remedy, determined by the way in which it is prepared. For first aid treatment the most commonly used potencies are 6C and 30C.

**Provings** Homoeopathic remedies are tested on healthy people. The symptoms they have after taking a remedy are the symptoms which that remedy will cure. These symptoms are written down in the Materia Medica, and are known as the provings.

**Remedies, Chronic** Deep-acting remedies used in the treatment of chronic disease, although at times they may act wonderfully well for acute ailments. There is a fine line between chronic and acute remedies.

**Remedy** What homoeopaths call their medicines. Remedies are most commonly in tablet or powdered form, although they can also be taken as a liquid.

**Succussion** The forceful shaking which, along with dilution, is part of the process of making a homoeopathic remedy.

**Suppression** Concealing of symptoms such as colds, skin eruptions and fevers can give rise to more serious systemic disorders. For example, the link between trying to suppress the skin eruptions caused by eczema and the development of asthma is well recognized by health practitioners (both orthodox and complementary).

**Susceptibility** An individual's unique response to disease. It is influenced by heredity and environmental factors.

**Symptom, Characteristic** A symptom that is peculiar, unusual and distinctive. It is not a symptom of the specific disease; it is a symptom that is unique to the sufferer. For example, a child with a very hot head, yet with cold hands and feet. These are also characteristic symptoms of the remedy *Belladonna*. Another example is a child who has a fever but who wants nothing to drink – this is an unusual, or characteristic, symptom.

**Symptoms, Emotional** A homoeopath will pay attention to the feelings patients have, particularly if they are too ill to guide the homoeopath to specific homoeopathic remedies which might be indicated for their physical problem.

**Symptoms, General** Symptoms that affect the whole person, not just the local part of the body that seems to be the focus of illness. A child will usually say, 'I feel ...' when talking about a general symptom, and 'My ...' when referring to a particular symptom. For example, if a child says, 'I feel much worse out in the cold air' or 'I feel better when I lie down', these are general symptoms. If a child says, 'My foot aches when I walk on it', this is a particular symptom.

**Symptoms, Mental** May reflect the inner self or the individuality of your child as shown on the mental level. Is he slow to learn? How is his memory? These symptoms are certainly used in constitutional or chronic treatment, and when obvious in acute situations will help when you are trying to choose the best remedy.

**Treatment, Constitutional** Aimed at the person's overall health, not just the acute episode of illness. When a child requires this type of treatment, you need to consult a qualified homoeopath.

**Vital Force** The elemental life-force, yet to be quantified by science. It is this vitality that we know as 'good health'. Homoeopathic remedies appeal to the vital force to promote self-healing.

# useful addresses

## UK

### HOMOEOPATHIC PHARMACIES

**Ainsworths Homoeopathic Pharmacy**
36 New Cavendish Street, London W1M 7LH
Tel: 020 7935 5330

**Helios Homoeopathic Pharmacy**
97 Camden Road, Tunbridge Wells, Kent TN1 2QP
Tel: 01892 536 393/537 254

**Goulds Homoeopathic Chemist**
14 Crowndale Road, London NW1
Tel: 020 7388 4752/387 1888

**G. Baldwin and Company**
171 Walworth Road, London SE17 1RW
Tel: 020 7703 5550

### FINDING A HOMOEOPATH

**British Homoeopathic Association**
27a Devonshire Street, London W1N 1RJ
Tel: 020 7935 2163
(send a sae for a list of doctors)

**The Society of Homoeopaths**
2 Artizan Road, Northampton NN1 4HU
Tel: 01604 621400

**The Society for Complementary Medicine**
3 Spanish Place, London W1M 5AN
Tel: 020 7487 4334

**Gabrielle Pinto**
Registered Homoeopath and Acupuncturist
Ms Pinto is based in London and can be contacted by writing care of:
The C. W. Daniel Company Ltd, 1 Church Path, Saffron Walden, Essex, CB10 1JP
*or*
e-mailing her at: gabrielle@fivebears.com

### FINDING A HERBALIST

**The National Institute of Medical Herbalists**
56 Longbrook Street, Exeter EX4 6AH
Tel: 01392 426 022

### PSYCHOTHERAPY AND COUNSELLING
You can either contact these places directly or write to the British Association for Counselling, which publishes a directory, at:
37a Sheep Street, Rugby CV21 3BX

**Anna Freud Centre**
21 Maresfield Gardens, Hampstead, London NW3 5SD
Tel: 020 7794 2313

**Institute of Family Therapy**
24–32 Stephenson Way, London NW1 2HX
Tel: 020 7391 9150

**Institute of Psychotherapy and Social Studies**
5 Lake House, South Hill Park, London NW3 2SH
Tel: 020 7794 4147

**Lincoln Centre and Institute for Psychotherapy**
77 Westminster Bridge Road, London SE1 7HS
Tel: 020 7928 7211

**London Centre for Psychotherapy**
19 Fitzjohns Avenue, Swiss Cottage, London NW3 5JY
Tel: 020 7435 0873

**Metanoia – Psychotherapy Training Institute**
13 North Common Road, London W5 2QB
Tel: 020 8579 2505

**The Minster Centre**
57 Minster Road, London NW2 3SH
Tel: 020 7435 9200

**The Westminster Pastoral Foundation**
23 Kensington Square, London W8 5HN
Tel: 020 7937 9355

### PREGNANCY, CHILDBIRTH AND POST NATAL CARE ORGANIZATIONS

**The National Childbirth Trust**
Alexandra House, Oldham Terrace, London W3 6NH
Tel: 020 8992 8637

**The Informed Parent**
19 Woodlands Road, Harrow, Middlesex HA1 2RT
*For information about immunization*

### BOOKSHOPS

**Ainsworths Pharmacy**
36 New Cavendish Street, London W1M 7LH
Tel: 020 7935 5330

**Helios Pharmacy**
97 Camden Road, Tunbridge Wells, Kent TN1 2QP
Tel: 01892 536 393/537 254

**Minerva Books**
6 Bothwell Street, London W6 8DY
Tel: 020 7385 1361
*Mail-order service available*

**Watkins Books**
19 Cecil Court, Charing Cross Road, London WC2N 4EZ
Tel: 020 7836 2182

## USA and Canada

### FINDING A HOMOEOPATH

**American Institute of Homeopathy**
1585 Glencoe Street, #44, Denver, CO 80220
Tel: (303) 370–9164

**Council for Homeopathic Certification**
P.O. Box 157, Corte Madera, CA 94976
Tel: (415) 389–9502

**Foundation for Homeopathic Education and Research**
2124 Kittredge Street, Berkeley, CA 94704

**International Foundation for Homeopathy**
2366 Eastlake Avenue East #301, Seattle, WA 98102
Tel: (206) 324–8230

**National Center for Homeopathy**
801 Fairfax #306, Alexandria, VA 22314
Tel: (703) 548–7790

**North American Society of Homeopaths**
Suite 350, 10700 Old County Road #15, Plymouth, MN 55441
Tel: (612) 593–9458

**Murray Feldman**
Vancouver Centre for Homoeopathy, 2246 Spruce Street,
Vancouver BC, V6H 2P3, Canada
Tel: (604) 733–6811

### SUPPLIERS
*Most of these suppliers also sell books about homoeopathy.*

**Boericke and Tafel**
2381 Circadian Way, Santa Rosa, CA 95407

**Boiron**
1208 Amosland Road, Norwood, PA 19074

**Dolisos**
3014 Rigel, Las Vegas NV 89102
*or*
1945, Boul. Graham/Suite 002, Ville Mt.-Royal,
Quebec H3P 1H1
Tel: (416) 764–0921 or (514) 735–3687

**Hahnemann Medical Clinic Pharmacy**
8828 San Pablo Avenue, Albany, CA 94706
Tel: (510) 527–3003

**Luyties Pharmacal**
4200 Laclede Avenue, St. Louis, MO 63108

**Standard Homeopathic Company**
204–210 West 131st Street, Los Angeles, CA 90061

BOOKSHOP

**The Minimum Price Homeopathic Books**
250 H. Street, PO Box 2187, Blaine, WA 988231
Tel: 1–800–663–8272, Fax (604) 597–8304

# further reading

Dr Margery Blackie, *The Challenge of Homoeopathy, The Patient not the cure* (Unwin Paperbacks, 1981)

Miranda Castro, *The Complete Homoeopathy Handbook* (Macmillan, 1991)

Catherine R. Coulter, *Portraits of Homoeopathic Medicines* (North Atlantic Books, 1986)

Paul Herscu, *The Homoeopathic Treatment of Children* (North Atlantic Books, 1991)

Dr Dorothy Shepherd, *A Physician's Posy* (The C. W. Daniel Company, 1981)

—, *The Magic of the Minimum Dose* (The C. W. Daniel Company, 1964)

George Vithoulkas, *Medicine of the New Man* (Thorsons, 1985)

## Childbirth and Child Development

Janet Balaskas, *New Active Birth* (Unwin Paperbacks, 1993)

Miranda Castro, *Homoeopathy for Mother and Baby* (Macmillan, 1992)

Judith Harris and Robert Liebert, *The Child: Development from Birth through Adolescence* (Prentice Hall, 1984)

R. Lansdown and M. Walker, *Your Child's Development* (Frances Lincoln Ltd, 1991)

Penelope Leach, *Baby and Child, from Birth to Age 5* (Penguin, 1979)

D. W. Winnicott, *The Child, The Family and the Outside World* (Penguin, 1957)

## Vaccination

Listed here are books, booklets and articles to help you find
information on the effectiveness and safety of vaccination:

Wallene James, *Immunization: The Reality Behind the Myth* (Bergin
and Garvey, 1988)

Leon Chaitow, *Vaccination and Immunisation: Dangers, Delusions
and Alternatives* (The C. W. Daniel Company, rev. edn 1998)

Department of Health, *Immunisation Against Infectious Disease*
(HMSO, 1992; issued to all General Practitioners)

Thomas McKeown, *The Role of Medicine* (Blackwell, 2nd edn,
1979)

Randall Neustaedter, *The Immunisation Decision: A guide for Parents*
(North Atlantic Books, 1990)

## Booklets

Dr Wolfgang Goebel, 'Should I have my child vaccinated?',
Anthroposophical Medical Association

Trevor Gunn, 'Mass Immunisation: A Point in Question' (Cutting
Edge Publications, 1992)

Lynn McTaggart (ed), 'The What the Doctors Don't Tell You
Vaccination Handbook' (Wallace Press, 1991)

R. D. Micklem, 'Measles: The Disease, the Vaccine, the
Homoeopathic Treatment' (available from Minerva Books – see
page 208 for address)

Committee on Safety of Medicines, 'Adverse Reactions to Measles
Rubella vaccine', *Current Problems in Pharmacovigilance* 21
(November 1995): 9–10

John M. English, *British Homoeopathic Journal* 84 (1995): 156–63

Richard Moskovitz, 'The Case Against Immunizations', *The
Homoeopath* 4.4 (1984): 114–41

—, 'Vaccination: A sacrament of modern medicine', *The
Homoeopath* 12.1 (1992): 137–44

Randall Neustaedter, 'Measles and Homoeopathic Vaccinations',
*The Homoeopath* 10.2 (June 1990): 31–2

—, 'Homoeopathic prophylaxis – is it valid?' *Resonance* Nov–Dec
1995: 12–14, 30

'A Shot in the Dark', *Sunday Times Magazine*, 17 December 1995: 17–23

(The three articles from *The Homoeopath* are available from the Society of Homoeopaths – *see page 206* for address.)

## Further Help

You may find it helpful to discuss the subject further with your homoeopath as well as your family doctor and health visitor. You may also wish to contact:

**THE INFORMED PARENT**
19 Woodlands Road, Harrow, Middlesex HA1 2RT

This is an organization established in 1992 by a group of parents which offers support and information to parents trying to decide about vaccination.

# bibliography

John Ball, *Understanding Disease* (The C. W. Daniel Company, 1987)

John Bowlby, *Attachment and Loss* (3 vols; Penguin, 1981)

Hamish Boyd, *Introduction to Homoeopathic Medicine* (Beaconsfield Pub. Ltd, 1981)

Miranda Castro, *The Complete Homoeopathy Handbook* (Macmillan, 1991)

Stephen Cummings and Dana Ullman, *Everybody's Guide to Homoeopathic Medicines* (Tarcher/Putnam, 1991)

V. Ghegas, *Classical Homoeopathic Lectures Volume C* (Homeo Study, 1987)

Chris Hammond, *How to Use Homoeopathy Effectively* (Caritas Healthcare, 1988)

Judith Harris and Robert Liebert, *The Child: Development from Birth through Adolescence* (Prentice Hall, 1984)

T. R. Harrison, *Principles of Internal Medicine* (McGraw and Hill, 9th edn, 1982)

Constantine Herring, *The Homoeopathic Domestic Physician* (Jain, 1993)

T. S. Iyer, *Beginners Guide to Homoeopathy* (Jain, 1992)

K. Kamal, *You and Your Child* (Jain, N.D.)

James T. Kent, *Repertory of the Homoeopathic Materia Medica* (Jain, 1987)

R. Lansdown and M. Walker, *Your Child's Development* (Frances Lincoln Ltd, 1991)

Robert Mendelssohn, *How to Raise a Healthy Child* (Contemporary Books, 1984)

*Merck Manual* (Merck, Sharp and Dohne Research Laboratories, 13th edn, 1977)

Roger Morrison, *Desktop Guide* (Hahnemann Clinic Publishing, 1993)

Randall Neustaedter, *Homoeopathic Paediatrics* (North Atlantic Books, 1991)

M. B. Panos & J. Heimlich, *Family Homoeopathic Medicine* (Orient Paperbacks, 1983)

Dr M. T. Sontwani, *Common Ailments of Children and Their Homoeopathic Management* (Jain, 1990)

# index

Page references in **bold** type indicate entries in the materia medica.